Chair Yoga Made Easy for Seniors Over 60

Step by Step Comprehensive Guide to Chair Yoga Made Easy for Seniors Over Sixty

Introduction

Do you desire an active lifestyle but fear that you may be unable to achieve it effectively at your age?

Are stiff joints preventing you from doing simple tasks that you used to do easily by yourself, and would you want to engage in easy exercises to become more flexible?

Are you considering chair yoga but would first want to know its ins and outs?

If you've answered yes, this book has been mindfully designed to give you an effective solution to all your troubles and worries above by teaching you the art of chair yoga.

Here, you will learn:

- The benefits of chair yoga to your health
- How to do chair yoga effectively
- The different safe chair yoga exercises that you can do
- And much more!

So let's begin!

PS: I'd like your feedback. If you are happy with this book, please leave a review on Amazon.

Please leave a review for this book on Amazon by visiting the page below:

https://amzn.to/2VMR5qr

Table of Contents

Introduction _____ 2

Chapter 1: History and Benefits of Chair Yoga _____ 6

Chapter 2: Safety Precautions When Practicing Chair Yoga _____ 9

Effective Chair Yoga poses for Seniors Over Sixty _____ 11

Chapter 3: Warm-Up Chair Yoga Poses ____ 12

    Breath Awareness _____ 12

    Warm-Up For The Spine _____ 20

    Warm-Up For The Fingers _____ 21

    Lower Body Chair Yoga Warm-Up Poses _____ 24

    Warm-Up For The Obliques and Spine _____ 27

Chapter 4: Upper Body Poses for Strength and Flexibility _____ 30

Seated Arms and Upper Body Workouts using Resistance Bands _____ 54

Chapter 5: Lower Body Poses for Strength and Flexibility _____ 66

Chapter 6: Core and Obliques Chair Yoga Poses _____ 83

Chapter 7: Cool Down Chair Yoga Poses _ 99

Conclusion _____ 102

Chapter 1: History and Benefits of Chair Yoga

Lakshmi Voelker first introduced chair yoga in 1982 as a solution for one of her students who had arthritis and was struggling with floor poses. It has grown in demand since then, especially because of its flexibility and inclusivity to the aging, injured, those with disabilities, and even office workers who spend over eight hours seated behind a desk.

The fantastic thing about chair yoga is that anyone can practice it, from kids to seniors.

Let us look at some benefits you are likely to enjoy by practicing chair yoga:

1. **Improved flexibility**

Your ability to make body movements such as bending, twisting, and stretching is essential for your everyday life, and being flexible will help you make such movements with ease. Chair yoga entails a regular range of motion to your tendons and muscles around your joints.

These motions improve your flexibility with time. The more flexible you are, the easier it gets to do everyday tasks.

Many people think that you lose flexibility as you age. While this may be true, flexibility is also something you can work on, and it is possible to be flexible while you age by being deliberate about it.

The fact that you're aging gives you an even better reason to be proactive and open to challenging yourself to improve your body flexibility.

2. Improved strength

You might be tempted to underestimate the power of gentle but regular body stretches because you feel you can only build your strength by lifting weights.

However, did you know that the contracting motions of muscles when doing chair yoga can actually build your strength?

Such gentle movements also improve your balance. When you have good balance, you reduce the chances of injuring yourself during workouts and will perform your daily tasks confidently without fear of hurting yourself.

3. Less stress and improved mental clarity

One thing with chair yoga and yoga, in general, is that you focus on your breathing and movements meditatively. This brings about mindfulness and harmony between the body and nature, which makes you relax, reducing stress and improving mental clarity.

Chair yoga, like other exercises, also improves your mood. When you exercise, your body releases endorphins, a body chemical associated with pleasure. Endorphins are usually produced when we indulge in pleasurable activities, making us feel good, improving our mood, and reducing our stress levels.

Actually, people who do regular physical activities have been known to be generally happier.

4. Better pain management

Many seniors over sixty battle osteoarthritis and other health complications. While there is no cure for osteoarthritis, chair yoga can help you manage the pain that comes with it and other health complications.

It diminishes pain by stretching those painful muscles and reducing chronic pain. When the muscles are stretched and the painful areas are hit, pain is eased.

5. Better sleep

Chair yoga is a meditative technique that calms and relaxes you. Once you are calm, it is easy to fall asleep. This is especially true when you do some yoga right before bed.

In cases where you do your yoga practice during the day, your muscles get tired from all the stretching and need to recover. Hence, you will notice that if you practice regularly, it will be easier for you to fall asleep, and you will start sleeping better and longer.

6. Affordability

Many people think they have to join some yoga class or community to practice yoga, which will cost them. While joining a yoga class wouldn't be a bad idea and is, in fact, a good motivating factor, it is also a choice.

The great thing about chair yoga is that you can practice it anywhere, at home or the office, using the available resources, such as chairs and guides such as this one, to help you maintain general wellness and good health. That is what makes chair yoga very accessible and flexible.

No expensive equipment is needed for you to do chair yoga - just you, some space, a chair, and motivation.

Chapter 2: Safety Precautions When Practicing Chair Yoga

While accidents happen all the time when people engage in physical activities, most of these accidents can be avoided by taking safety measures before and during sessions.

So before we look at the different chair yoga poses, your safety is important whether you are a beginner, have some medical limitations, or are even a pro yogi. The following safety precautions will prevent injuries or painful experiences during your chair yoga practice:

1. **Stay aware**

Pay attention to your body before the workout to evaluate what feels good and what to avoid.

Red flags such as headaches and dizziness should not be ignored because they could signify that you need medical attention first. A physical therapist or your doctor will be able to advise you accordingly.

2. **Chair positioning**

Your chair should be stable, without arms to help you perform different poses, and with a straight back. Place the chair on a flat surface for more stability.

In cases where you feel that the floor is slippery, have the chair on a yoga mat to prevent it from slipping and causing injuries to you.

3. Warm-ups

Warming up is essential. It prepares your body for physical activity, increases or ensures blood and oxygen flow into your muscles, and prevents injury by increasing your muscle temperature.

4. Dressing

Wearing proper workout attire is also important when practicing chair yoga. You should wear light activewear that will allow you to stretch easily. When you wear comfortable clothes, you won't have to worry about discomfort and will therefore focus on yoga and not on what's keeping you uncomfortable.

5. Go slow

It is important to progress at a pace you feel comfortable with during chair yoga. Do not attempt to move too fast or try poses that don't feel stable for you, as doing this can easily lead to injury.

Over time, as you become more flexible, stable, and have better balance, you can do the poses comfortably, so be patient with yourself.

Next up, let's dive into the exercises!

Effective Chair Yoga poses for Seniors Over Sixty

The chair in Chair Yoga is used for support. You can have a variety of poses, seated on the chair, standing, or any other position, but using a chair for support.

In chair yoga, you will be coordinating your breathwork with your physical activities throughout the practice. This is because yoga is a mind, body, and spiritual practice that aims to harmonize physical and breathing techniques to ensure your general well-being.

This section will teach you breath-awareness and how to incorporate it into the various poses that you will do:

It is critical to note that you do not have to spend a lot of time practicing yoga; just a few minutes, like 30 minutes or even less, is all the time you need to notice results.

I have categorized the yoga poses in this book into:

- Warm-Up Poses
- Strength and flexibility poses
- Cool down Poses

Let us start with chair yoga poses for warming up your body.

Chapter 3: Warm-Up Chair Yoga Poses

I mentioned warming up as a safety precaution before getting into your practice session. The warm-up should take only five to ten minutes of your yoga session to get your body ready.

You can choose any of these warm-up poses. Try and balance them so that at the end, you will have worked all the major parts of your body, from your head to your toes.

Let us get started:

Breath Awareness

Breathing is a big part of yoga. You need to start by grounding yourself by bringing your attention to your breathing. You breathe all the time, but the times you focus solely on your breathing are minimal.

In yoga, noticing how you breathe helps you be in the moment and mindfully connect with yourself, your surroundings, and the present moment. This can help prevent injuries because you are aware of what is happening.

Deep breathing

- Sit upright on your chair and make yourself comfortable. Your back should be long and straight, shoulders aligned with your hips, head high and straight up.

- Pay attention to how the air comes in and goes out through your nose. Take in a deep breath and hold for two seconds, then exhale to release.

- Repeat and observe your belly expanding and relaxing and air coming in and out through your nose. Become aware of your environment, then your breathing.

Throughout your yoga session, try to apply this breath awareness technique by breathing in and out through the nose to help soothe your nervous system.

Breathing Hands Rub

- Take both of your hands and rub them together to generate some heat. Start gradually and slowly increase your speed. Coordinate your breathing with your hands.

- Bring your hands to the center, palms together, and then pull them apart just a little and bring them back to the center.

- Breathe in as you pull your hands apart and out as you get them back to the middle. Repeat five times.

- Place your hands together, and now, instead of pulling them apart to the side, pull your right hand diagonally towards the ceiling and your left hand diagonally towards your knees, and then bring them back to the middle.

- Breathe in as you pull apart and out as you bring them back to the middle. Repeat this five times and return to the starting position.

Breathing seated cat-cow pose

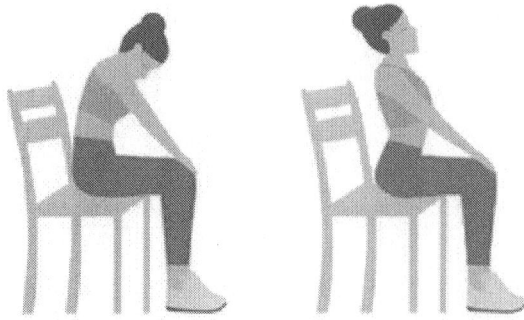

- Sit upright with your spine neutral and shoulders aligned with your hips. Begin with the cat pose.

- Place your hands on your thighs and elongate your spine. Draw your belly inwards towards your spine and the spine towards the back of your chair, and exhale.

- Then do the cow pose by inhaling while you relax your belly, move your shoulders backward and your head up to face the ceiling. Push your spine towards your belly. Please note that the cat pose rounds your back and spine while the cow pose works the opposite way. Continue with the flow from cat to cow poses, five times for each.

Breathing Shoulder Rolls

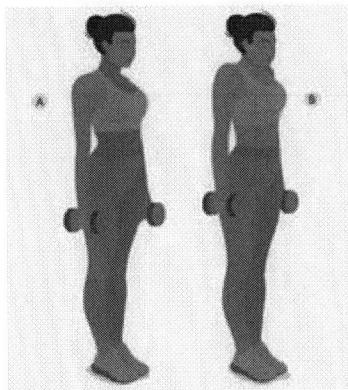

- Start by sitting upright with your shoulders aligned with your hips and your head straight.

- Breathe in while you roll your shoulders forward and up. Do not be tempted to lean backward or forward. Then breathe out while you roll your shoulders backward and downwards and relax.

- Repeat the same pose, shoulders up and forward as you breathe in, then downwards and backward as you breathe out and relax.

- Repeat this ten times.

Breathing Chair Yoga Shoulder Shrugs

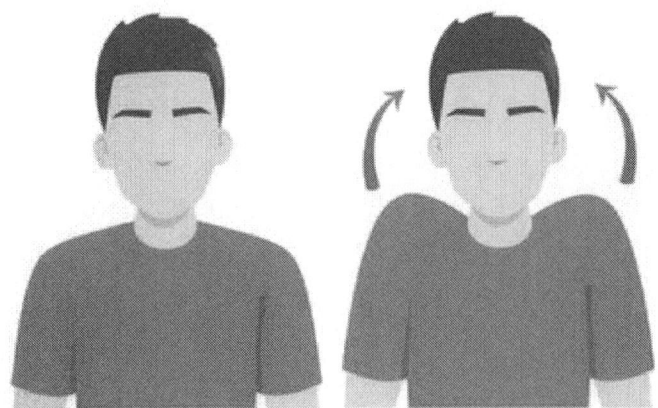

- Sitting upright on your chair, ensure that your spine is neutral.

- Squeeze your shoulders together as you inhale and lift them towards your ears.

- Release your shoulders to return to the original position and exhale and relax. Repeat ten times.

Breathing Seated Chair Yoga neck stretch

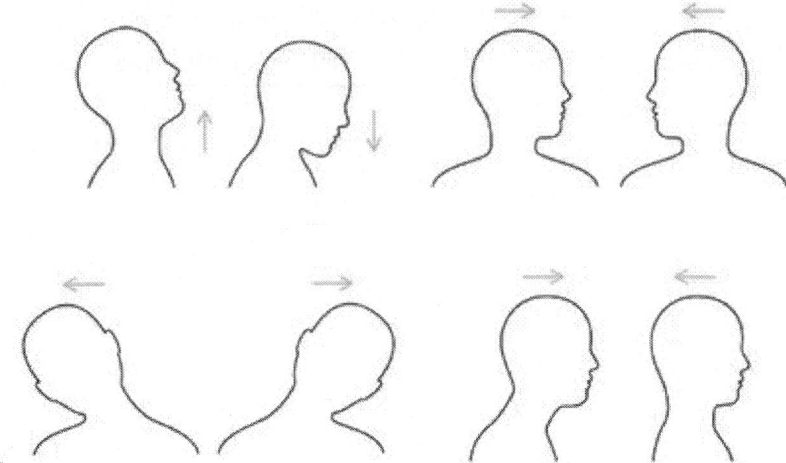

There are several poses that you can do to stretch the neck.

- To start off, ensure that you are seated upright with your spine neutral and shoulders in line with your hips.

- Slowly drop your chin towards your chest and try not to move your shoulders; lean forward, not backward.

- Now lift your head up slowly up to the point where your face will be facing the ceiling. Drop your head again slowly and back up. Repeat this ten times.

- Bring your head back to the center, and slowly tilt your neck to have your head facing to your right side, your chin directly above your right shoulder, and your face on the right side.

- Gently move your head back to the center and then to your left shoulder so that your chin is directly above your left shoulder. Try not to move the rest of your body, but just the head.

- Repeat this ten times.

- This time, with your head at the center, begin to circle it so that you start at the center with your chin facing your chest, then lift your head towards the left and back to the center to face the ceiling. Then move towards the right and back to the center with your chin facing towards your chest again.

- One complete circle is one repetition. Inhale when you move towards the left, and exhale when you move towards the right side. Repeat this ten times

- While still sitting upright with a neutral spine, head at the center, place your hands on your thighs, and ensure that your head is straight up.

- Gently move your head up as if lifting your left ear towards the ceiling, tilt your head towards your right shoulder, and then relax.

- Gently move your head up again, lifting your right ear towards the ceiling, and then tilt it towards the left shoulder and relax for a second. Inhale when moving to one side, and exhale as you move to the other side.

- Repeat this ten times for each side.

To intensify this, when tilting the head side to side, use your hand to pull your head gently towards the shoulders for extra sensation. Use the right hand when moving your head towards your left shoulder and your left hand when moving your head towards your left shoulder.

- Now, in the same neutral spine position and head centered, this time move your head and nose towards your right armpit. Have your right hand at the back of your head and gently pull towards your armpit.

- Move your head back to the center and move your head and nose towards your left armpit. Use the left hand to pull your head gently from the back towards your armpit.

- Inhale when you move to the right, and exhale when moving your head towards your left armpit. Repeat this pose ten times for each side.

You should feel a stretching sensation from the top of your neck, back, and shoulder blade.

Warm-Up For The Spine

The following stretches will help warm your spine up and prepare you for the real thing.

- Sit tall on your chair with your spine neutral and your head up high.

- Open your legs wide. This time, your center is your chest and not your head.

- Gently lean your chest towards your right knee. No need to go all the way down; lean close to the knee but don't actually touch the knee.

- Slowly return to the center, and lean your chest towards your left knee.

- Get close but do not touch it, and then return to the center. Inhale as you lean towards the knee and exhale as you return to the center.

- Repeat this five times.

- After the fifth time, in the next repetition, make a complete circle by leaning slowly towards your left knee, and instead of moving back to the center, move across to your right knee and back to the center.

- Inhale as you complete the circle, and exhale when you relax at the center. Repeat this pose five times.

Warm-Up For The Fingers

You also need to allow blood and oxygen to flow to the fingers. Stretching the fingers will help you, especially if you have stiff fingers.

Wiggling and stretching fingers

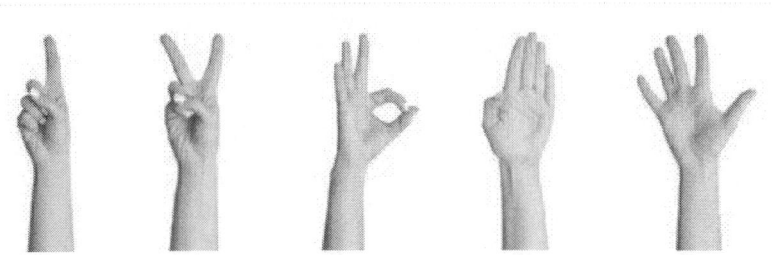

Straighten your hands and lift them to your chest level, then begin to wiggle your fingers as if counting them one by one. When done counting all the fingers, wiggle all of them together at the same time. Do this for thirty seconds.

You can also fold your fingers into a fist still from the same position, holding for two seconds and releasing with ten repetitions.

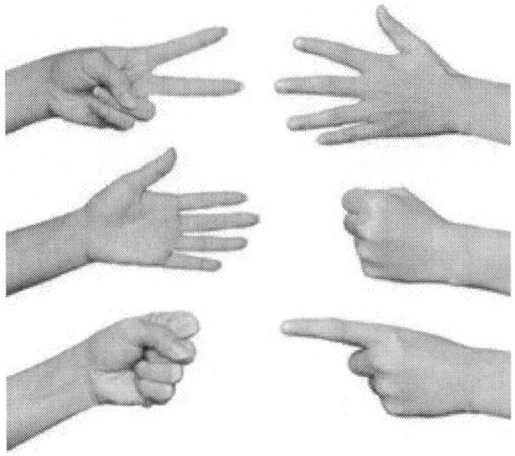

Now with your hands hanging in the air, wag your palms like a dog would wag its tail. Let your hands be free, and do this for twenty seconds.

Hand stretching warm-up

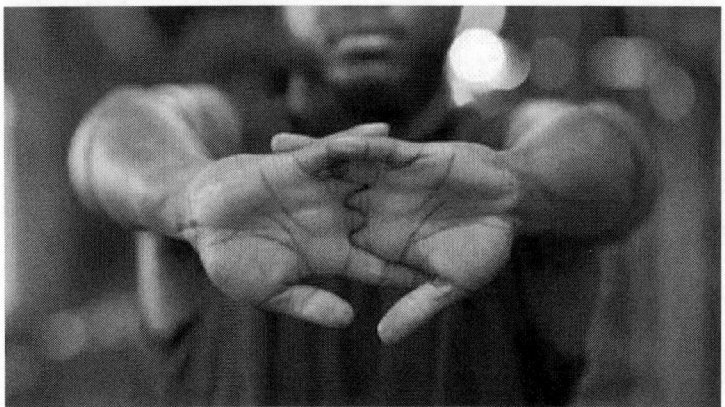

- Bring your hands together and interlock the right-hand fingers with the left-hand fingers. Hold them that way near your chest, and then extend them forward in front of you.

- Once you have reached the maximum stretch, turn your palms to face outside and the back of your palms to face you. Feel the stretch on your hands.

- Hold for twenty seconds and relax.

Lower Body Chair Yoga Warm-Up Poses

To warm up your lower body, do the following exercises:

Light leg slaps

- Begin to slap your thighs with both hands lightly – light, quick taps moving from the top of your thighs to the inside and the sides moving down to your legs.

- Try to tap the accessible parts of your back thighs as well.

This allows blood to circulate down to the thighs and the legs.

Ankle rolls

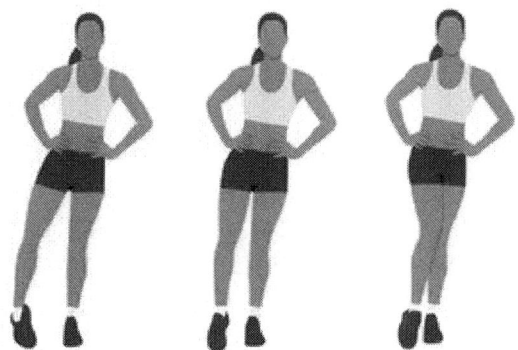

- Try and sit at the tip of your chair, but ensure that you are stable and safe. Then extend one of your legs forward, your toes up, and your heel on the ground. If you feel strong enough, lift your leg slightly off the ground. If not, it's still fine on the ground.

- Move your toes to touch the ground as you inhale, and then lift the toes to face up so that your heel now touches the ground. Switch to the other leg and repeat the same motions. Repeat ten times for each leg.

- If your leg is slightly lifted off the ground, move your toes gently to face up and then gently have them face forward. Repeat ten times for each leg.

- Now make circular motions around the ankle, moving your foot from the right and completing on the left side. Do this ten times for each leg.

Seated Groin stretch

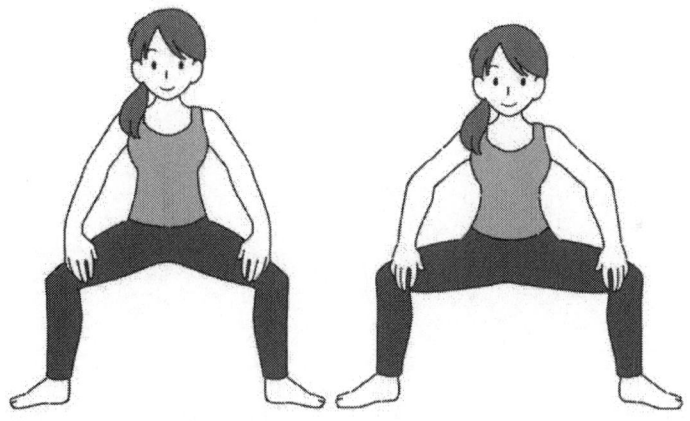

- Sit on the chair with your back neutral. Keep your legs wide apart, then bring your head slowly downwards to face the ground.

- Move your elbows toward your inner thighs and gently push your inner thighs outwards using your elbows.

- Feel the stretch on your groin, inner thighs, core, shoulders, and back .and then relax. Inhale as you push your inner thighs with your elbows and exhale when you relax.

Warm-Up For The Obliques and Spine

Seated Side Bend

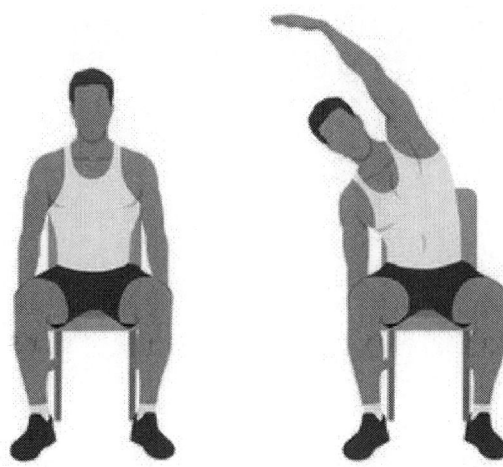

- Sit upright on your chair with your spine neutral.

- Hold your seat with your left hand on the left side, and slowly shift your weight to the left arm.

- Lift the right hand up to the ceiling, then move it towards the left side. Feel the stretch on your obliques. Inhale as you stretch to the left. Slowly return to the center.

- Now hold the right side of the chair with your right hand and shift your weight to your right arm. Raise your left hand to the ceiling and bend it to the right side over your head. Exhale as you stretch to the right.

- Repeat ten times, and then relax.

Spinal twist

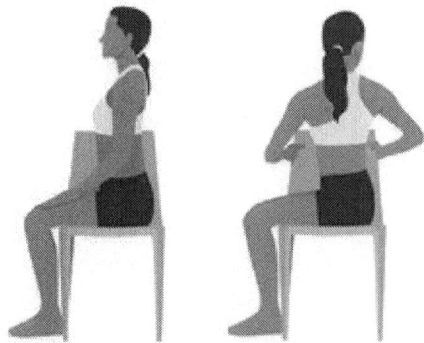

- The spinal twist is meant to warm up your back and spine, allowing blood circulation to your back.

- Sit facing one side of your chair, right or left. Your spine should be neutral. Raise your arms to your chest level and twist your upper body towards the chair. Your upper body should remain upright.

- Return to the original position and repeat. Inhale as you twist towards the chair and exhale when you return to the starting position.

- Face the other side of your chair. If you were facing the right side, now switch to the left. Sit with your spine neutral, then twist your upper body to face the chair. Inhale as you turn to face the chair and exhale as you relax.

- Repeat this ten times.

These warm-up chair yoga poses can also be performed during the main session, but you will do them for longer than when warming up.

You can choose any of the poses, but do not spend more than ten minutes here unless that is all you intend to do for that session.

Chapter 4: Upper Body Poses for Strength and Flexibility

Now that we are warmed up and blood and oxygen are nicely flowing throughout the body, let's proceed to the next poses that will strengthen your muscles and make your body more flexible.

These poses have been categorized according to the body part they target.

- Upper body
- Lower body
- And core

This chapter focuses on upper body exercises:

Eagle arms

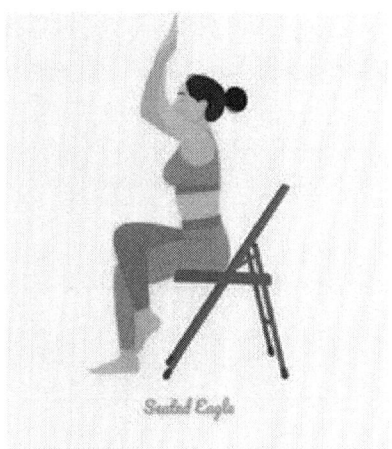

- Extend arms straight in front. Cross your arms with your right arm under your left arm. Wrap your elbows together and cross your hands again at the wrist. Hold that pose for three to four breaths.

- With your hands locked together like that, lift your elbows up gently as you inhale. Lift until you cannot lift them any further, and then bring them down. Exhale as your elbows come down.

- You will feel the stretch under your left shoulder. The higher you lift your arms, the more the sensation. Repeat this twenty times.

- Relax your hands. Shrug your shoulders up and down, extend them again in front of you, and cross them, this time with your left arm under your right arm. Wrap your elbows together and your wrist together as well. Then lift your wrapped arms to the furthest point that you can go. You will feel the stretch on your right arm.

- Inhale as you lift your elbows and exhale as you lower them. Repeat this twenty times.

The regular eagle arms pose also involves crossing your thighs together, as in the image above. This is a more sensational version of chair yoga if you wish to go for a more challenging pose.

Gentle Chair Yoga Twist

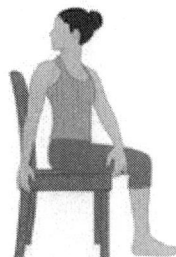

- Sit tall with an elongated spine, feet on the ground, and your head up, facing straight ahead.

- Place your arms on your lap, your right arm on the left lap, and left arm on the right lap.

- Release the right arm and move it behind you on the chair. Turn your upper body to face the back, chin above your right shoulder. Breathe in as you twist towards the back.

- Relax and return to the initial position with your arms on your lap. Remember to cross your arms so that the left arm is placed on the right lap and vice versa.

- This time release the left arm and have it behind you on the chair. Turn your upper body to face the back with your chin above the left shoulder.

- Inhale as you face the back and exhale as you return to the starting position. You will feel a stretching sensation on your spine, shoulders, obliques, and even your hands if you stretch them correctly.

- Repeat this ten times for each side. Alternate the twists between the right and left sides; one twist to the right and one twist to the left counts as a complete repetition.

Seated Child's pose

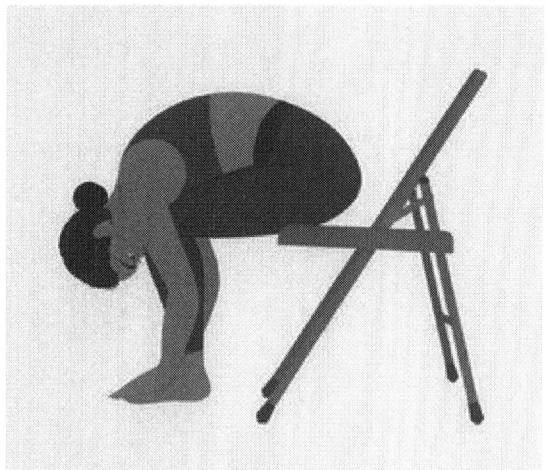

- Sit tall, your spine extended, your hands free, and your legs slightly apart. Slowly bend forward towards your thighs, your hands dropping towards your feet and tucking your head in between your knees.

- Breathe in as you bend and hold for a second. Come back up to an upright and extended spine position slowly as you breathe out. Repeat five times.

Extended Side Angle Pose

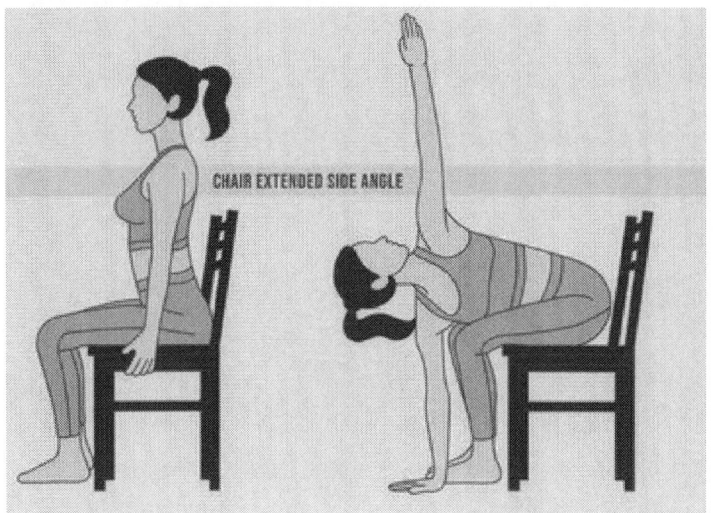

- On your sixth rep of the seated child's pose, have your left arm touch your right foot, then slowly lift your right arm and head towards the ceiling so you are facing the ceiling and your right arm is lifted up towards it.

- Breathe in as your lift your right arm. Hold for two seconds and return to the starting position.

- Switch to the other arm. Have your right hand touch your left foot and lift your left arm and your head to face the ceiling. Inhale as you move up. Hold for two minutes.

- Feel the stretch on your shoulder, obliques, and neck. Hold longer if you want to feel the stretch more. Repeat ten times.

Sun Salutations

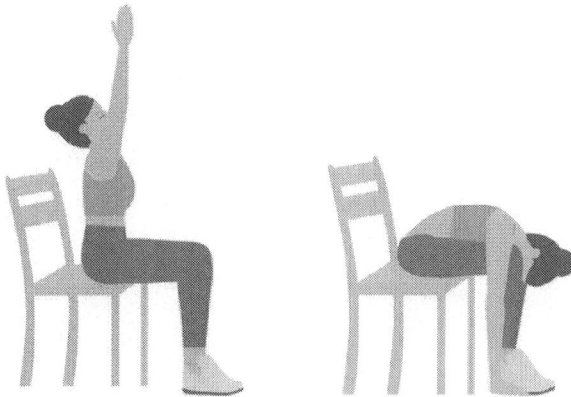

- After your fifth repetition of the child pose, return your hands to your feet, and tuck your head between your knees.

- Slip the back of your hands against the floor and gently raise them up towards the ceiling as you slowly lift your upper body to a seated position.

- Inhale as you lift yourself to sit. Hold for two seconds and slowly lean forward and down to your thighs, hands towards your feet on the floor.

- Exhale as you move towards the floor.

- Repeat ten times and relax.

Sideward Reach

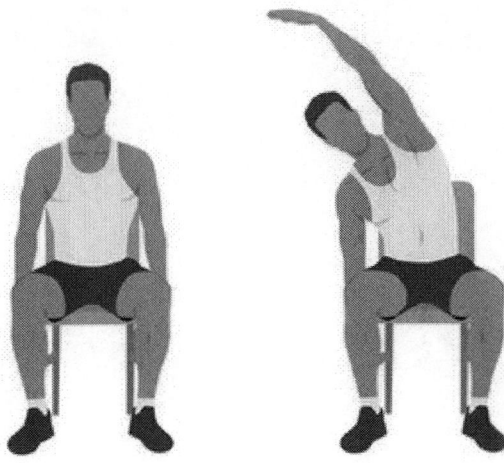

- Sit tall on your chair. Have your right hand hold the left side of your chair for support.

- Lift your left hand towards the ceiling and over your head towards the right side. Here you will be stretching the hand and the obliques. Breathe in as you extend your hand to the right and hold for two seconds.

- Now repeat with the right arm. Have your left hand hold the right side of your chair across your laps, and then lift your right hand over your head to the left side.

- Breathe in as you stretch your right hand. Hold for two seconds then return to the initial position.

- Repeat ten times.

Reverse Arm Hold

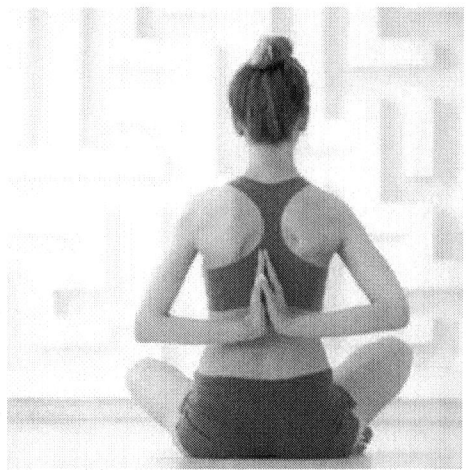

To do the reverse arm hold, sit and maintain your spine in a neutral position.

- Stretch both of your arms to the sides to meet behind you and hold, as shown in the image above - opposite hand to touch opposite elbow.

- Squeeze your shoulder blades backward and release both the shoulders and your arms. Inhale as you hold your arms together and exhale as you release.

- If it's difficult for you to touch the elbows, have your opposite hand hold the hand part of the other arm. Strive to feel the stretch.

- This exercise stretches your arms, back, and shoulders.

The reverse arm hold is very similar to the Reverse Namaste pose. Instead of holding your arms together, your palms will meet behind your right hand and left-hand fingers.

This stretch isn't easy, and therefore do not despair if you do not get it right the first few times; as you get flexible, it will get easier to do, and as long as when you do it you feel the stretch, it will still be effective.

Seated Warrior 1 Chair Yoga Pose

There are different modifications to the Warrior 1 pose. You can try both and go with the one that feels more comfortable and effective to you, or if they're both good for you, you can do them interchangeably.

Variation One

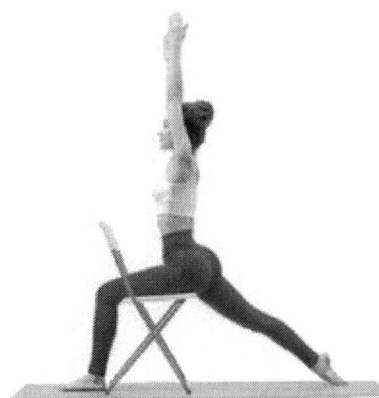

- Sit upright on your chair, facing the right side of the chair. Step the right foot forward, and the left foot (the foot at the edge of the seat) should step back.

- Lift your arms up slowly.

- Push your left leg back up to the point where you feel the stretch on your core and your hand up to the point where you feel the stretch on your arms and shoulders. Hold for two seconds and relax. Inhale as you move the hands up; exhale as you relax.

- Switch to the left side of the chair and repeat the same move. Do five repetitions for both sides. If you like to intensify the warrior 1 pose, make the repetitions ten for each side.

Variation two

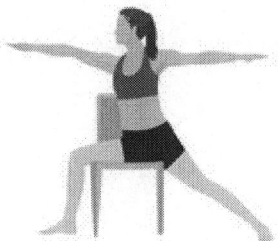

- Still in the same position, one leg bent at the knee and the other stretched behind you, stretch your arms sideways to open your chest, forming a cross.

- Open them wide enough, and ensure you do not lower them at any point. Inhale as you open your arms. Hold for two seconds and slowly return them to hug yourself tight as you exhale.

- Squeeze that hug and feel the stretch on your shoulders and neck. Repeat this ten times and relax.

Variation three

- Return to the original position and bring your elbows and palms together in front of you. Lift the elbows the furthest that you can lift them.

- You will feel the stretch at the back of your shoulders and triceps. Inhale as you lift your elbows. Lower your elbows to a Namaste pose with your palm together in front of you, like in a prayer.

- Repeat this five times.

On the sixth repetition,

- Lower your elbows in front of you. With your arms still bent at the elbows, move them to the side to open your chest wide. Open to the furthest point as you can go.

- Inhale deeply as you open. Slowly bring the elbows together right before your chest as you exhale.

Variation Four

The fourth modification is a little easier than the first.

- Sit facing forward with a straight back. Inhale as you lift your arms up to meet above your head. You can even clap and immediately lower your arms to face the floor as you exhale.

- Repeat ten times.

- If you want to enhance the intensity of this, extend to twenty repetitions.

- This warrior 1 pose stretches your core, shoulders, arms, and legs.

Seated forward bend

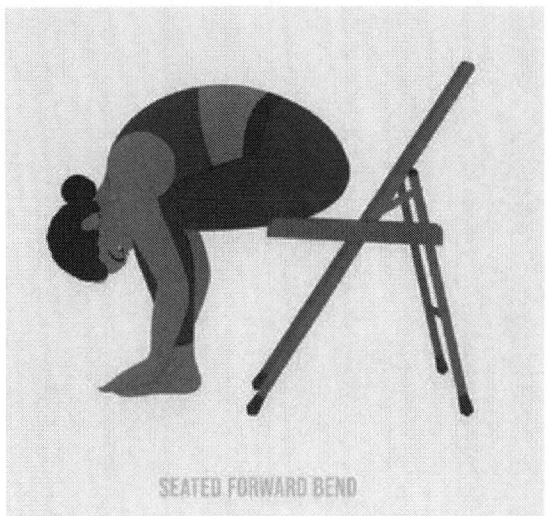

- Sit at the edge of your chair having the spine extended. Ensure that you are steady enough so that you do not fall. Bring your feet together.

- Rest your palms on your thighs and bend forward towards your thighs to tuck the head between your knees.

- Squeeze your shoulders back and as you tuck your head closer to your knees, squeeze until you feel the stretch on your triceps, the back of your neck, and your back. Take a deep breath as you bend.

- Slowly go back to the original position as you exhale. Repeat ten times.

You might notice the similarities with the sun salutation. The only difference is the positioning of your arms.

Dips

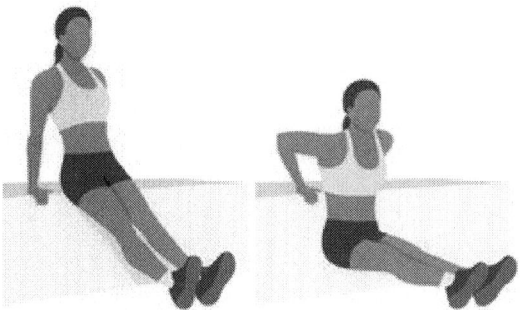

Dips will help strengthen your chest and triceps. Dips lean toward some of the challenging chair yoga poses for the upper body. Therefore, if you feel it's too difficult, skip to the next pose.

Let us see how to do dips properly:

- Sit tall on your chair with your hands firmly holding the chair by the sides fingers facing forward, as in the image above. Your knees should be bent, and your feet soles on the ground.

- Begin to walk forward so that the chair is behind your butt, and you are hinged at the waist and knees.

- Lower your upper body for your hips to come close to the ground. How low you go depends on your fitness level, then lift yourself up to the chair level. Within the third repetition, you will feel the stretch on your triceps.

- Exhale as you move your upper body to the ground and inhale as you lift yourself up.

- Repeat ten to twenty times.

To make dips more challenging than they are,

- Sit tall on your chair and straighten your legs in front of you, to have your heels on the ground.

- Move your hips away from the chair, leaving your hands to support you on the chair. The difference with the first dip is the position of your legs.

- Begin to lower your upper body towards the floor in a slow and controlled way. Come back to the chair level when you get close to the floor

- Inhale as you lower your body and exhale as you lift your body up again.

- Repeat ten to twenty times

To break the monotony of seated poses, let's look at some standing yoga poses. Just stand and move behind your chair for this.

Standard standing yoga pose

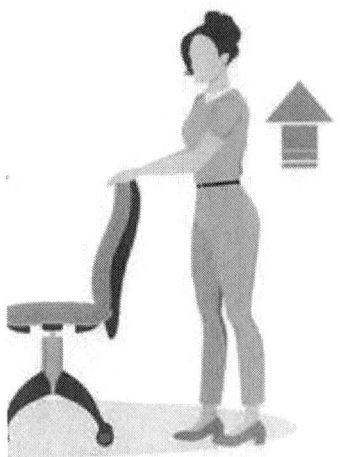

- Start by warming up the feet and ankles. Put your feet close together, both knees and ankles.

- Have your ears over the shoulders, back nice and tall, elongated spine, pelvic neutral such that it does not lean forward nor backward, and your neck straight.

- Lift your heels to place weight on the toes. Lower them to have your weight on the soles of your feet and lift yourself back up on your toes.

- Hold the back of your chair for support.

This can also be done in reverse.

- Put your weight on your heels, and ensure an elongated spine, straight back, and shoulders over your wrists.

- If necessary, hold the back of your chair for support.

- Begin to lift your toes for your weight to be pushed over to your heels. Lift both toes simultaneously and consciously as you take deep breaths. Do this twenty times.

- Now alternate left leg to right leg. Lift your right leg toes as you inhale and lower them as you exhale. Lift your left leg toes as you inhale and lower them as you exhale. Continue to twenty repetitions.

- This warm-up pose will strengthen and make your ankles flexible as well as help you with good posture and balance

To add a variation to this, lift one heel while the other is on the ground. Bring the lifted heel down, lift the other one, and keep alternating them until you can feel the stretch on your ankles and the back of your legs.

Standing Chair Yoga Lunge

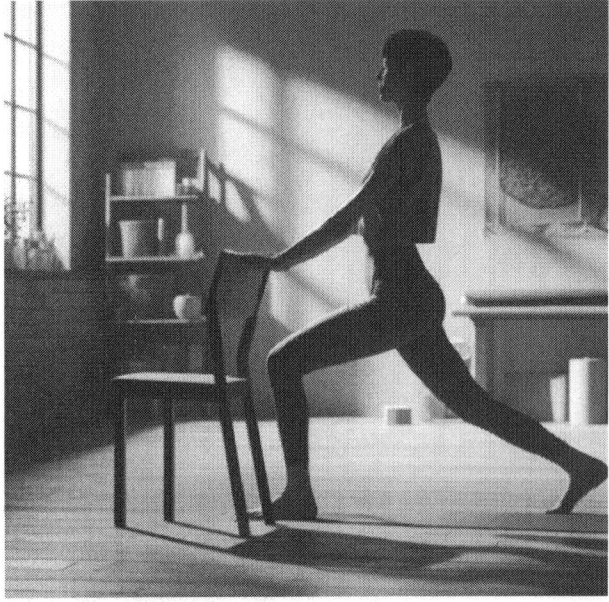

Stand behind your chair, bring the right foot forward and extend the left foot behind you. You can choose to have your heel raised or have your foot sole on the ground, bend your right foot knee to go into a lunge position, holding the chair for support.

- Keep your spine nice and tall, and straighten your left leg behind you. You will feel a stretch on your core and lower back.

- Take your right arm and lift it towards the ceiling. Inhale as you take your hand up. Hold for three seconds.

- Lower your hand back to the chair as you exhale, and then lift the left hand as you inhale; hold for three seconds and keep alternating the hands in ten to twenty repetitions.

- Switch legs to have your left foot forward and your right foot extended behind you, keeping your back nice and tall. Begin to lift your arms towards the ceiling, holding for three seconds as you take deep breaths and as you alternate your hands.

- Repeat ten to twenty times for each

With your feet still apart, move the chair further in front of you to prepare for the next pose.

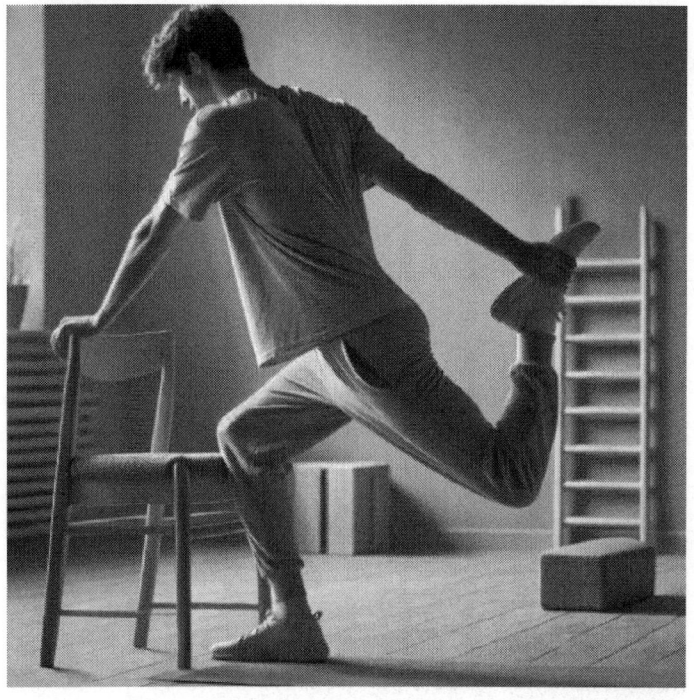

- Hold the chair with both of your hands, lean the elbows as you lean forward towards the chair without moving your feet.

- With your right foot forward, slowly lift your left foot behind you as if trying to level it with your butt, but it does not have to be on the same level as you inhale. Feel that stretch sensation on your core and lower back. Keep the raised leg straight and hold for two seconds.

- Lower the left foot close to the ground but don't touch the ground; lift the foot back up behind you.

- If you want to challenge yourself, stretch your left arm in front of you, lift your foot higher or circle your ankle behind you.

- Lower your foot and then change your legs to have your left foot forward, right foot stretched out behind, arms stretched out to hold the chair in front of you, and your chest and head leaning towards the chair.

- Lift your right foot behind you as you take deep breaths and hold for three to five seconds. Lower it close to the ground and lift it again, just like you did with your left foot.

- Stretch your right hand in front of you as you support yourself with your left hand on the chair.

- Repeat ten to twenty times for each leg.

The Standing Cat-Cow Chair Yoga Pose

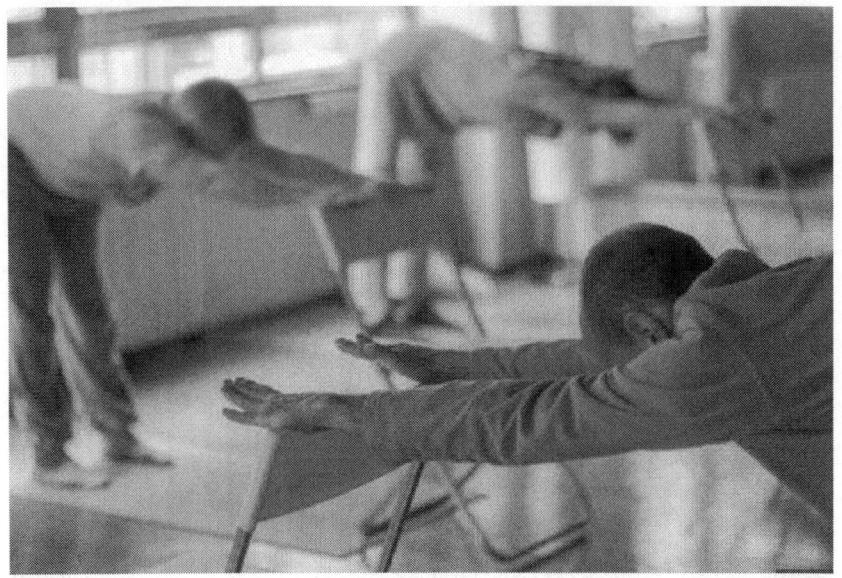

Earlier, we did the seated cat-cow pose during warm-up. The concept is the same as the standing cat-cow chair yoga pose, but you will be standing behind your chair this time. The standing cat cow yoga pose stretches your back, chest, and neck.

- Grab the back of your chair and walk backward away from the chair.

- Begin by inhaling and performing the cow pose. Walk your feet apart and bend your knees slightly.

- Lift your face slowly and look forward. Your belly button moves outwards while the lower back is pulled in.

- Exhale as you slowly lower your chin to tuck it and the tailbone between your arms. Your belly should be pulled in, and your back should be pulled out.

- Repeat ten to twenty times.

Side Angle Pose

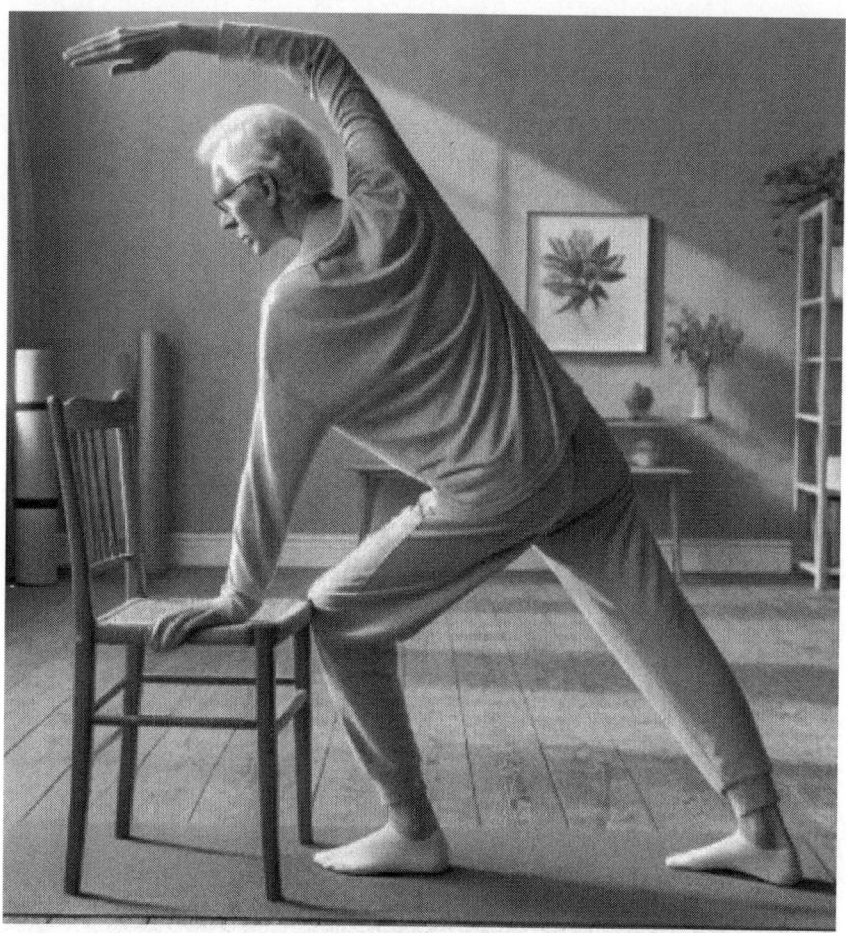

- Stand beside the chair, on the right side, back nice and tall. Bring your right foot to rest on the chair while the left foot stays on the ground.

- Rest your right elbow on your right lap. To feel the stretch on your hips and waist, lean slightly forward.

- Lift the left hand above and have your gaze follow your hand. You will be able to feel a sensation at the back of your shoulders. Hold for five seconds and relax. Repeat ten to twenty times.

- Move to the left side of the chair, and have your left leg resting on the chair.

- Bring your left elbow to rest on your lap. Lean slightly forward to feel the stretch on your left hip.

- Lift your right hand towards the ceiling to feel that stretching sensation at the back of the shoulders.

- Repeat ten to twenty times.

Seated Arms and Upper Body Workouts using Resistance Bands

For the following poses, you will need a resistance band as a prop to nail these poses successfully.

Resistance bands are easy to use and great for beginner yogis, those recovering from an injury, and even seniors.

You can buy a workout resistance band, or you can use a strong and elastic fabric, although we'd recommend the workout resistance band because it's been designed for this.

The poses below will increase your strength, mobility, and flexibility. And what's more, these poses are fun to do.

You can totally skip those poses that you feel are too challenging for your fitness level.

Seated resistance band pull-apart

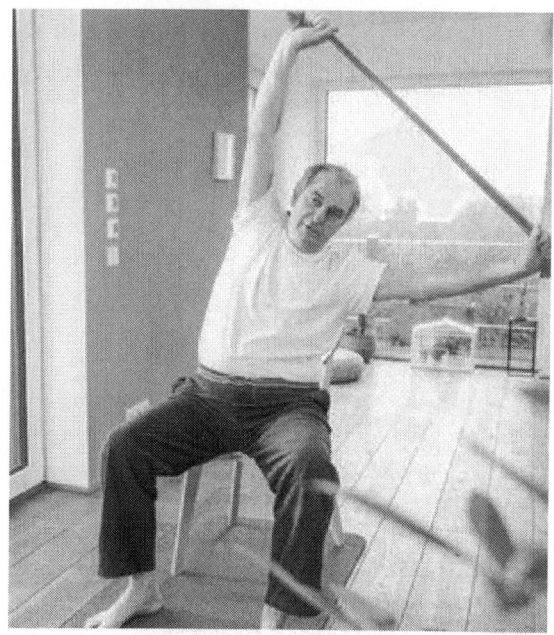

- Sit on your chair with a straight back and feet on the ground.

- Hold both ends of the resistance band to your chest height. The closer your hands are to the resistance band, the harder the resistance and the harder the stretch will be. If you are just beginning, give yourself a larger allowance between your hands.

- Engage your breathing and move your hands apart to bring the band to your chest, on your nipple line. Avoid the common mistake of moving the chest closer to the band. Only your hands should move.

- Relax your hands and repeat. Give yourself minimal breaks, and repeat ten to twelve times in one to two sets.

Pull-aparts can also be done from behind your back. This is what I mean:

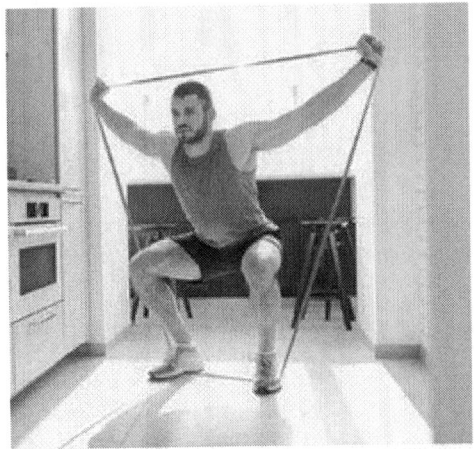

- While holding your resistance band as though you are ready for another repetition, lift your hand over your head. Now instead of having the band come close to your chest, when you pull the band apart, it will pass behind you to just below your shoulders.

- Repeat ten to twenty times.

Seated Overhead Resistance band Stretch

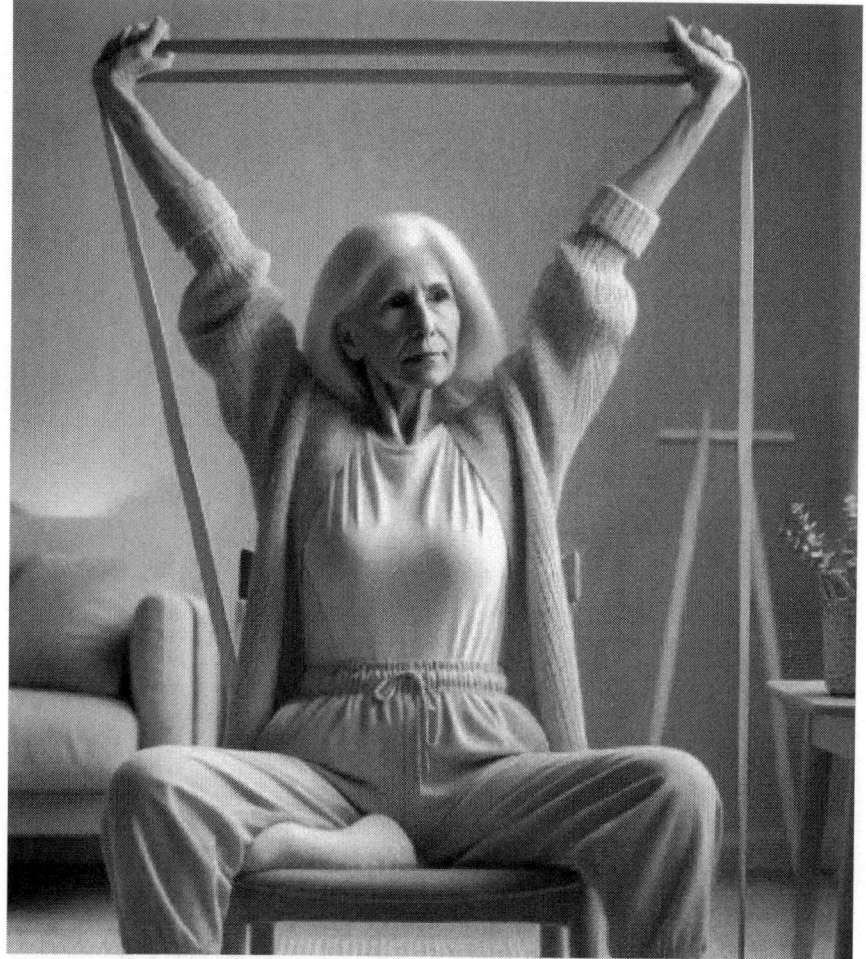

- Sit on the chair with your back nice and tall, your feet on the ground, and your hand holding two points apart in the resistance band, just as you did earlier with the seated resistance band pull aparts.

- You should be able to feel some resistance in the band. The resistance you want will depend on your strength and fitness level. If you are a beginner, minimal resistance will be manageable for you.

- Lift your hands over your head. That is where you will feel most resistance, then drop your hands behind you so that the resistance band comes behind you to the hip height.

- Remember to inhale as you move the band over your head to the back behind you.

- Lift your hands back from your hips, over your head, and on your laps in front of you.

- Exhale as you return your hands to the front.

- Repeat ten to twenty times in one to two sets.

- Avoid shrugging your shoulders and hardening your stomach the whole time you are doing this pose.

Also, avoid moving your chest or chin. Stay tall and neutral. Seated resistant

Band Bicep Curls

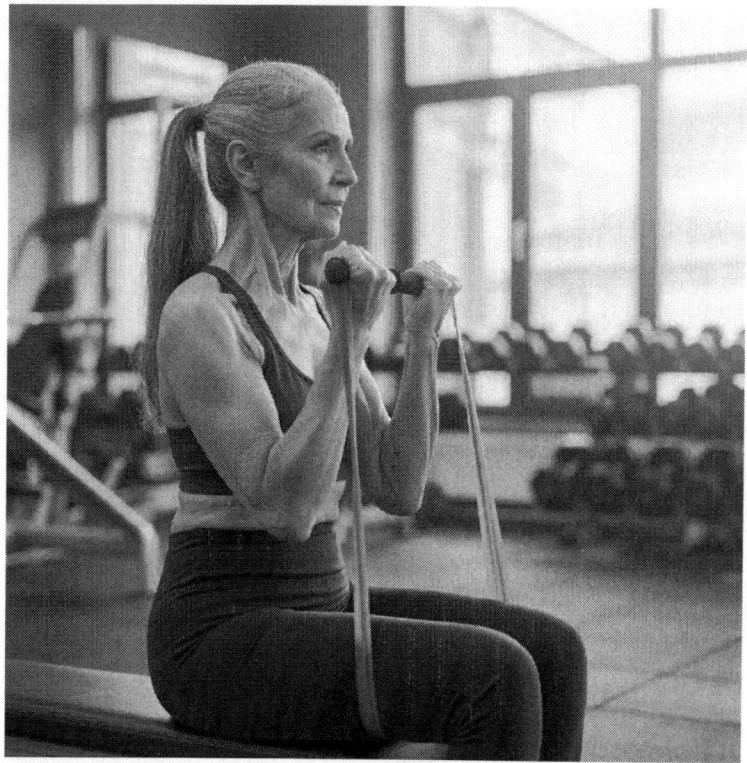

- Sit tall on the chair having your feet on the ground.

- Hold each end of the resistance band with your hands. Drop the resistance band to the floor, and step on it to have it pass below your feet, as shown above. This will cause some resistance on the band.

- Pull the band towards yourself from both ends, ensuring that you do not bend to meet it. Let the band move towards you.

- Inhale as you pull the band towards you.

- Slowly drop your hand towards your feet as you exhale.

- Repeat ten to twenty times.

To make this more challenging, drop your band on the ground and cross the ends with opposite hands. This will tighten the band more. And then, you can repeat the steps above.

- After the last repetition, return to the original position where you were seated tall on your chair, with your band passing below your feet.

  This time, we will work the biceps one at a time.

- Starting with the right hand, relax your left hand and pull your right hand to straighten it to the side while still holding the band. The resistance on the band here will stretch the bicep and shoulder muscles.

- Slowly drop your hand next to your hips facing the floor and immediately pull the band again, just as you did with the first pull.

- Repeat ten times and give the right hand a rest.

- Using the left side now, and still holding the resistance band, pull the left hand to straighten it to the side.

- Inhale while you pull and exhale as you return your hand down.

- Repeat ten times.

Another variation to the seated resistance band bicep curl is that instead of pulling the band towards you, you pull it sideways, lifting your hands straight beside you in ten repetitions.

The Overhead Press

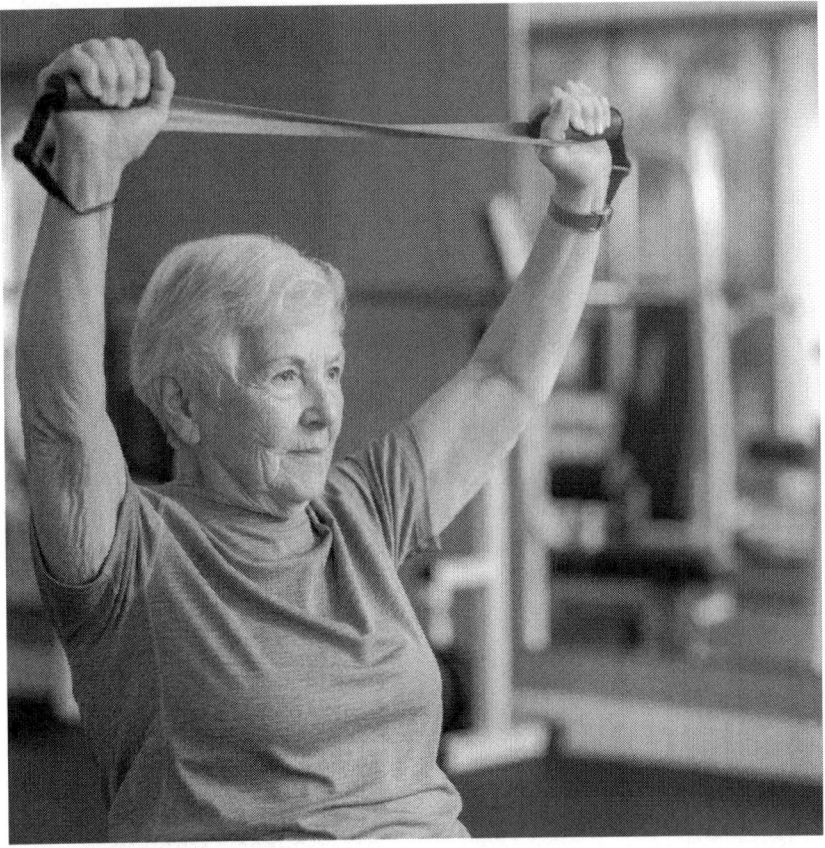

- Sit on the chair in the same position you were in when you did the bicep curls, your back tall and feet on the ground.

- You can have the resistance band pass under your chair, or you can sit on it like in the image above.

- Hold the ends of the band and pull it up and behind your arms.

- Pull the resistance band up towards the ceiling with both hands, aiming to straighten your arms. It is fine if you do not have them fully straightened up; as long as you feel the resistance as you pull up, it will still be effective.

- Inhale as you pull and exhale as you relax.

- Repeat ten times.

You can modify this pose

- In the same original position with the resistance band behind your arm, lift each arm alternating left to right as you stay keen on your breathing

- Repeat ten times for each arm.

Triceps resistance band kickback

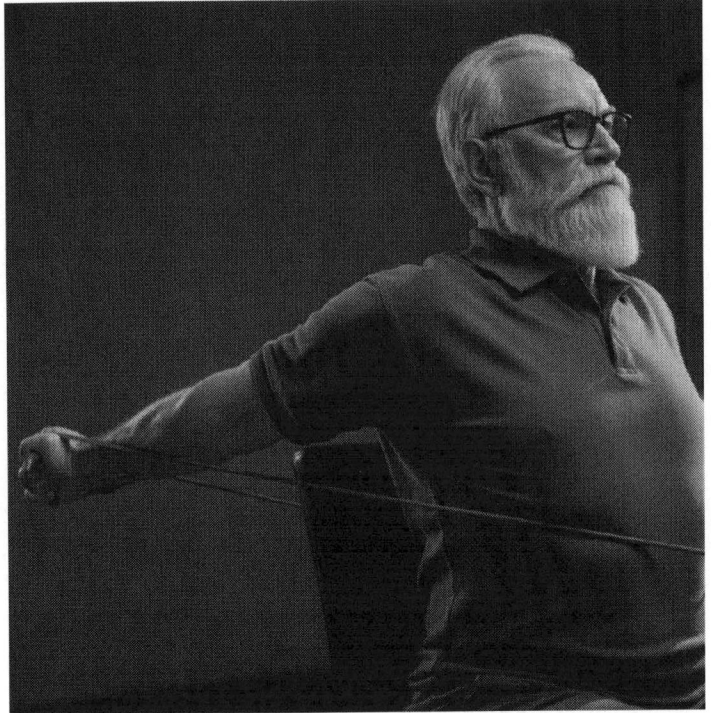

The triceps kickback will stretch and strengthen the triceps muscles.

- Grab any point of the resistance band with your left hand near one of its ends. Make sure to leave enough allowance for the kickback.

- Hold the other end of the resistance band with your left hand.

- Place your right hand on your left lap, still holding onto the resistance band.

- Pull the band back using the left hand as you feel that resistance on the band.

- Bring the hand back in and pull it back again.

- Inhale as you pull your hand back and exhale as you bring it in.

- Repeat ten to fifteen times.

- Change hands to have the left hand hold any point of the band and your right hand to hold the end.

- Begin to pull backwards just as you did on the other side, as you feel the stretch on the triceps.

- Repeat ten to fifteen times.

Chapter 5: Lower Body Poses for Strength and Flexibility

Most lower body poses target the hips, glutes, hamstrings, legs, ankles, feet, and in some cases, the core (abdomen).

You can use props such as a belt, a strong piece of cloth, or a strap as a hack for some poses to make them workable.

Seated Glute Stretch

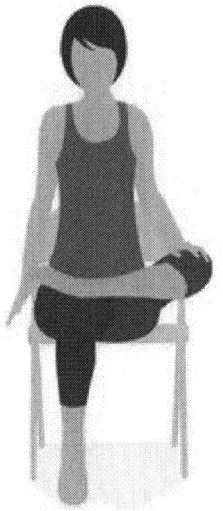

- Sit at the chair's edge with your back straight and spine extended.

- Bring your right foot on your left thigh and then lean forward to a position that is comfortable for you. You can use your hands to hold the leg in place. You can also intensify the stretch by placing your right-hand elbow on the right-leg knee. Take deep breaths as you hold for five seconds.

- Drop the right leg and repeat with the left leg. Lift your left leg, rest it on your right thigh as you take deep breaths, and lean forward. Hold for five seconds and release. Try up to three repetitions.

- Depending on your flexibility and comfort, you can make your hold shorter than five seconds.

If it is difficult to lift your leg to rest on your other leg's lap, use a block to lift it at least one or two inches higher. Then place the side of your leg on the block (See the image above) to feel that stretching sensation on your hips and glutes.

Seated Squat

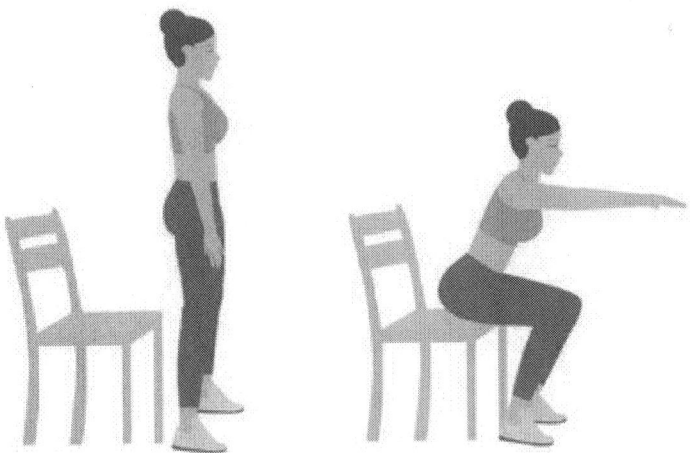

- Start by squeezing your glutes together as you release five times, to warm up your glutes.

- Sit at the chair's edge with your spine neutral and your legs slightly apart.

- Try to keep your knees pushed out because you will notice that they will keep getting pushed in.

- Extend your arms straight in front of you. They will help you keep balance as you get off the seat.

- Get off the chair, squeeze your glutes and sit back on the chair. You can stand all the way up and then sit down. Inhale as you stand and exhale as you get back on the chair.

- Repeat ten times and relax.

Hamstring Stretch

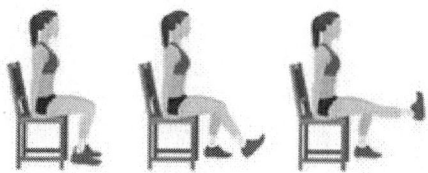

For this pose, you can use a strong long piece of cloth, a belt, or a strap as a prop. The goal is to touch your toes with your fingers, which can be a challenge to many senior yogis. So to make it manageable, you will use the belt or a piece of cloth to try and reach your foot.

- Sit close to the edge of the chair with both feet on the ground.

- Hold both ends of the belt or the piece of cloth with your hands to form a loop, and then insert your right foot into the loop, as in the image above.

- Hold your seat with one hand for support if needed while the other hand holds the belt.

- Pull the leg towards you without bending it at the knee. Pay attention to the stretch on your glutes and hamstrings. In this case, it's okay if you cannot completely straighten the leg, so long as you feel that stretch on your hamstrings. Ensure also that you keep your back straight.

- Take deep breaths as you pull your leg towards you using your prop of choice. Hold for five seconds and switch to the left leg, and repeat.

Hamstring stretch variation

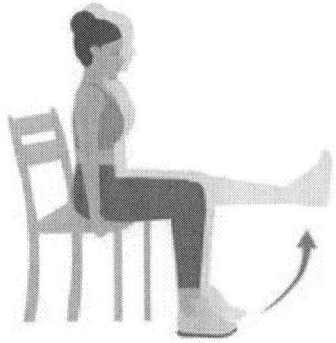

This is a modification to the hamstring stretch. You might need a block to raise your leg higher for extra comfort.

- For this pose, move to the edge of the chair, keep your back straight and spine neutral.

- Extend one foot forward and have the back of your heel on the floor while your other foot is bent at the knee and the entire foot is on the ground.

- Bend forward, maintain a straight back, and feel the stretch on your hamstring. To modify this to be less intense and to make it easier, you can add a block on the floor to bring your foot higher from the ground.

- Hold for five seconds, take deep breaths, switch to the left leg, and repeat.

Seated Hero Pose

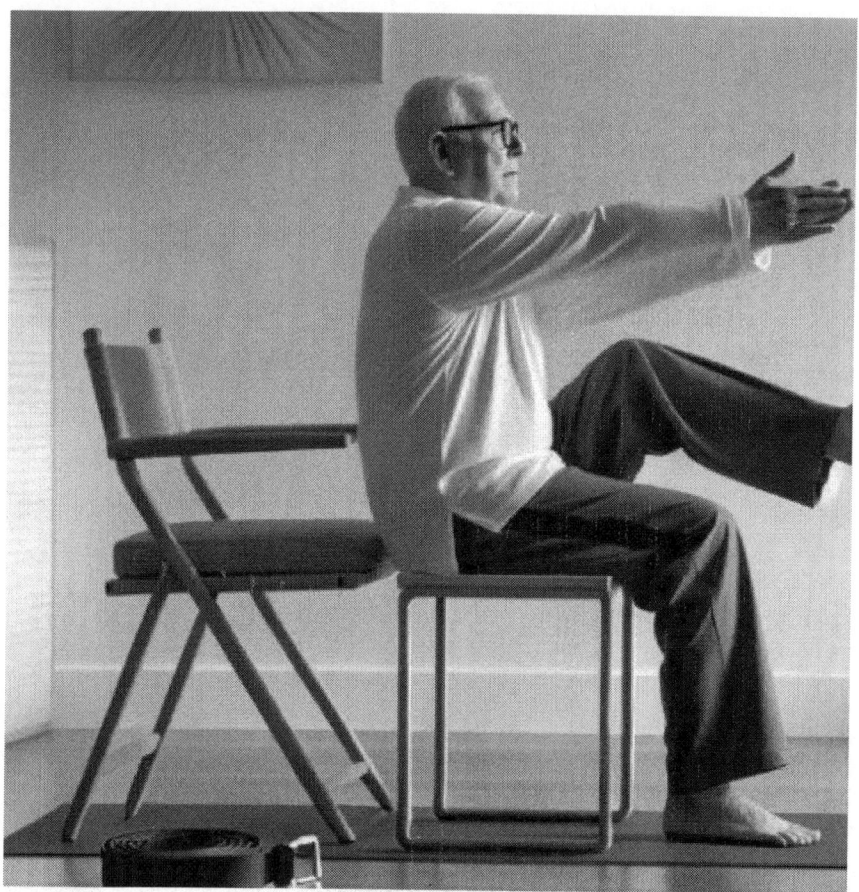

- Move to the right side of your chair, almost like you're sitting on one butt, and hold the chair on the left side with your left hand to add extra support. Move to the furthest end of the chair for more stability.

- Bend your left knee to ninety degrees and step on the ground with your toes.

- Hold your right foot with your right hand behind you and pull the heel towards your butt.

- Lean forward with a straight back to feel the sensation on your hip flexors and quadriceps.

- Discontinue the pose if you feel the stretch sensation on your knee because that is not normal. The seated hero pose targets the front part of the thigh and hip flexors.

- Hold for five seconds as you take deep breaths and release.

- Switch to the left leg and repeat.

- To make it easier to hold your leg behind you, you can use a belt, a strap, or even a strong piece of cloth like we did in the Hamstring stretch.

- The more you bend forward, the more sensation you will feel.

Seated Leg Raises

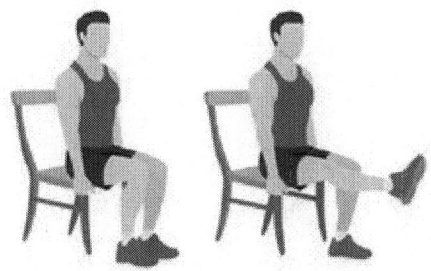

The seated leg lifts strengthen the muscles around your knees and quadriceps

- Sit on the chair with your knee bent at ninety degrees. Raise the right leg slowly and straighten it at a hundred and eighty degrees. Hold for five seconds keeping the left leg bent at ninety degrees.

- You can grab the sides of your chair with your hands for extra support. Make sure to keep your back straight for good posture.

- Slowly bring the right foot to the floor as you exhale.

- Switch up the legs to have the right knee bent at ninety degrees, then slowly straighten and raise your left foot and hold just like you did with the right foot. Hold for five seconds and repeat five times.

- Stand at the chair's side, holding the side of the chair for support with your left hand.

- Slowly lift your right foot and place it on the chair and load your weight on the left foot.

- Inhale and as you exhale, begin to hinge yourself at the hips as you place your left forearm on the back of your chair. Bring the right hand to your right lap.

- You can take your left hand from the back of your chair to reach the seat. Notice the stretch on your right hip.

- Take your right hand and lift it towards the sky to open your chest. Hold for five seconds and bring your hand back to the hips. Repeat ten to twenty times.

- Bring your right hand back to the hips, place your left hand back on the back of the chair, and slowly lift your upper body to stand up. Lower your right foot to the ground and switch sides.

- Move to the other side of the chair.

- Bring your left foot to the chair seat, and begin to hinge at the hips as you take deep breaths.

- Lean forward and place your left forearm on the back of the chair. Feel the stretch on your left hips.

- Lower your right hand to touch the seat, and lift your left hand towards the ceiling as you open your chest. Hold for five seconds and relax. You will feel stretching at the back of your shoulders and hips.

- Repeat ten to twenty times.

After the repetitions, return your right hand to the back of the chair and the left hand to your hips, and then lift your upper body to stand back up.

Chair Lunges

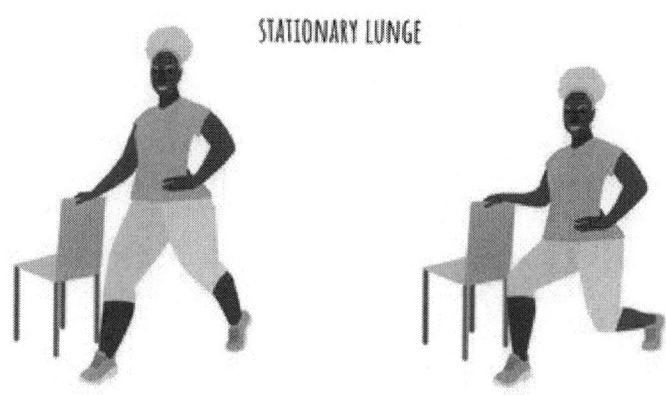

Chair lunges are to be approached with caution. Lunges in general, are challenging enough, and you could easily injure yourself if you do not do them cautiously.

In this case, the lunges you are about to perform have been modified to suit seniors and beginners.

You will need props such as a firm stick. It can be a walking stick or a broomstick. The other prop you will need will be a pillow placed on the chair for a soft landing.

- Sit at the edge of the chair facing the right side so that your right leg is bent 90 degrees at the knee and the sole of your foot is on the ground.

- The left foot is almost kneeling but does not actually touch the floor and is supported on the ground with the toes. Refer to the image above.

- Hold on to the stick with your left hand while your right hand is holding on to the chair for extra support.

- Have your back straight, place your weight on your right foot and lift yourself to stand as you inhale.

- Lower yourself down to sit on your right butt and immediately lift yourself up again.

- Do the lunges slowly as you pay attention to your breathing. After five to ten repetitions, turn around and do it on the left side.

- Sit at the edge of the chair facing the left side, left leg bent 90 degrees at the knee, sole on the ground, and the right leg almost kneeling on the ground but supported by the toes.

- Place your weight on the left foot and lift yourself to stand.

- Slowly lower yourself to sit and repeat five to ten times

You can start slow, say five to ten repetitions on the first day, and then do it twice a week, not necessarily every day until you are confident that you can perform the lunges comfortably.

Hip Thrusters

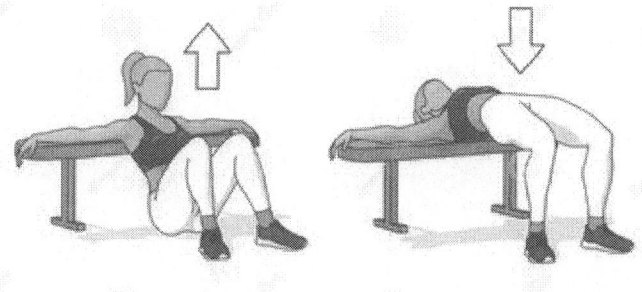

Hip thrusters will work your hip, glutes, and core.

You can place the chair next to the wall for more stability.

- Sit on your mat, leaning next to the chair. Lift your knees and move your toes close to your butt.

- Place your upper body on the chair for support.

- Press through your heels to push your hips to lift them up. You might need to walk your feet forwards just a little. Lift to the point where your back is straight, pelvic area is neutral, and your head is in line with your hips.

- Your head should not be dropping backward but remain aligned with the rest of your body.

- Hold for two seconds then lower hips without touching the floor. Stay in that position for two seconds and lift back up.

- Engage your breathing; inhale as you lift and exhale as you lower your hips.

- Repeat ten to twenty times and relax.

Chair Crunch Kicks

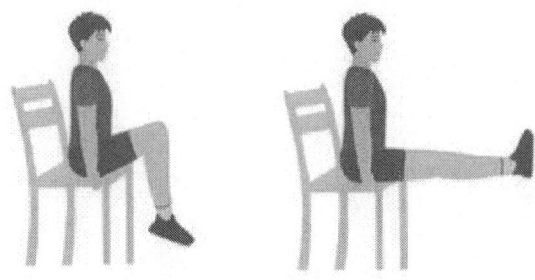

Chair crunch kicks are a powerful core and thigh pose. However, they can be very challenging, especially if you are just beginning. So you can start with a few repetitions several inconsecutive days a week and then increase the number of repetitions as your flexibility improves.

- Sit on the chair, press your back on the seat and bring your hands behind the chair to hold it firmly for support.

- Raise your legs up, bend the knees while your legs are still raised.

- Slowly kick forward with your feet to straighten them in front of you.

- Bring your feet back to the bent knee position.

- Strive to Maintain your feet raised and avoid curving your back until you are done doing ten repetitions.

- Inhale as you bring your feet towards you and exhale as you kick.

- Repeat ten times.

Side-to-side knee sweeps

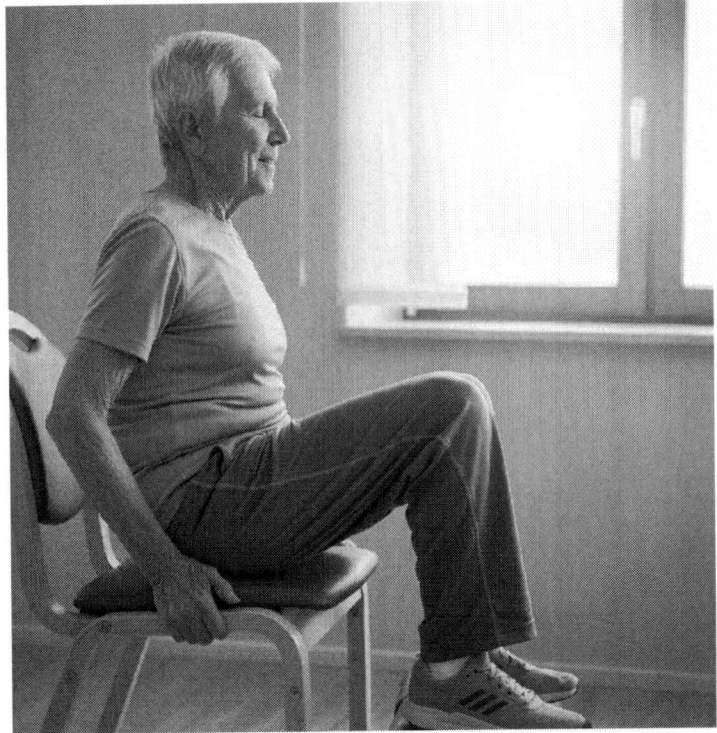

- Sit at the edge of the chair, grabbing it by the sides. Ensure your back is straight.

- Lift your feet off the ground and fold them at the knee. Lean back slightly and harden your core.

- Begin to slide your knees right to left while still bent.

- Take a deep breath as you move side to side and exhale as you return to the middle.

- Repeat ten times in two sets.

Triangle Pose

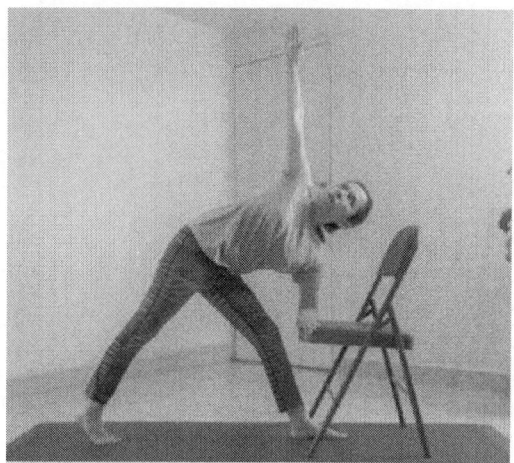

- Stand facing the chair and then step the right foot back, facing the right side, while the left foot remains facing forward. The left leg should be right under the foot of the chair. Have your legs wide apart.

- Bend to rest your hand at the edge of the chair with your left hand to stretch your hips and obliques.

- Lift the right hand towards the ceiling and hold for three seconds. Take deep breaths as you stretch. Gaze up at the lifted hand.

- Repeat the stretch ten times, switch to the left side, and repeat the same moves.

- Stand in front of the chair, move the right foot forward and left foot behind you, and move the legs apart until they are both straight.

- Bend forward to place your elbows on the chair and your head to face the chair.

- Feel the stretch on your left hip. Hold for five seconds and relax. Take a one-second break and repeat with the same left leg ten times.

- Relax and stand straight. Now have your left foot forward and your right foot behind you.

- Hold the chair with your hands and bring your elbows to the chair.

- Ensure that your legs are apart and straight, and feel the stretch on your right hip as you take deep breaths.

- Repeat ten times as you did with the first leg.

Chapter 6: Core and Obliques Chair Yoga Poses

We have looked at poses that strengthen the upper and lower body. You might notice that the core kind of gets stretched in the process, even though the poses do not really target the core. But what poses can you do to stretch and strengthen your core specifically? These poses have been highlighted for you in this chapter:

Abdominal Squeeze

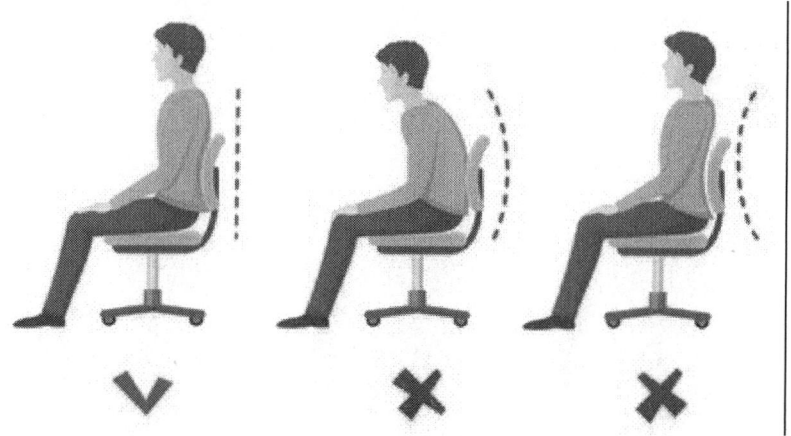

- Sit on the chair and make yourself comfortable, with your back straight and spine neutral, knees bent at ninety degrees.

- Harden your abdomen and draw it in as you inhale. Hold for four to five seconds and release. Exhale as you release.

- Repeat in three sets with twenty repetitions on every set.

Pay attention to the stretch on your stomach, and move at a controlled pace.

Boat Pose

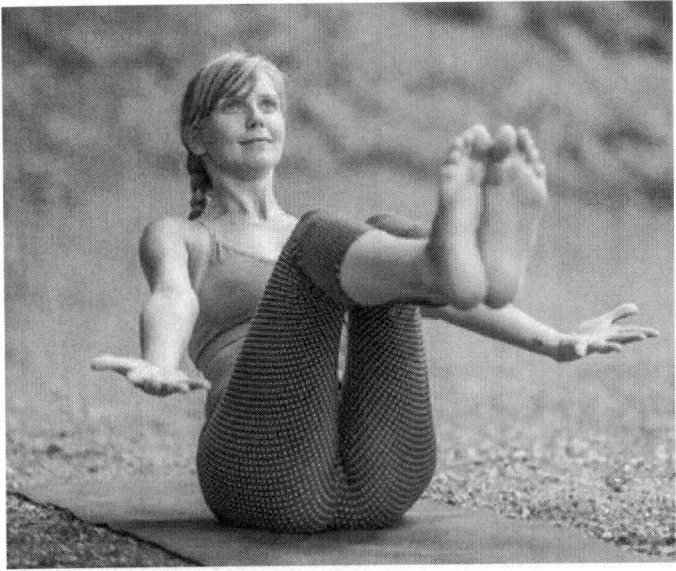

- Sit steady at the edge of the chair, and hold the sides with your hands for support.

- Press your knees together and begin to lift them towards your chest. Try your best to keep your back straight. Inhale as you lift your knees to your chest.

- Once you have gained some stability in that position, release your arms from the chair and spread them apart to open your chest.

- Bring your arms parallel to each other in front of you and hold in that position for two seconds as you engage your abdomen.

- Lower your feet to the floor, and bring your hands slowly to the ground as you bend forward for a forward bend to complete one repetition. Tuck your head between your knees.

- Start again by lifting your hands slowly over your head and then release them to hold the sides of the chair and repeat the boat pose. Repeat this five times.

You can also involve your legs to modify the standing chair yoga cat-cow pose. This one will have more sensation on your core which is the target.

- On your eleventh repetition, as you lift your head towards the sky, extend your right leg up and behind you as you inhale.

- Hold for two seconds and slowly bring it back towards your chest as you do the cat pose so that your knee and head move towards the chest as you exhale.

- Repeat ten times and switch to the left leg. Make the same moves with the left leg and repeat ten times as well.

Modified Mountain Climbers

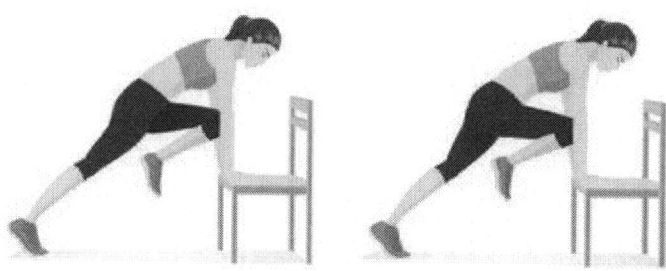

- Grab the sides of your chair firmly, as in the image above. Assume a plank position with your back straight, spine neutral, and your shoulders aligned with your wrists.

- Lift your right leg, draw your knee towards your chest, and slowly extend it back.

- Alternate from right to left leg as if climbing a hilly place.

- Repeat ten times for each leg. Move slowly to give yourself time to feel the sensation on your core.

- Inhale as you draw each knee in, and exhale as you extend it back behind you.

Besides strengthening your core, mountain climbers will also make your flexors strong and flexible and the obliques strong.

Chair Yoga Plank Pose

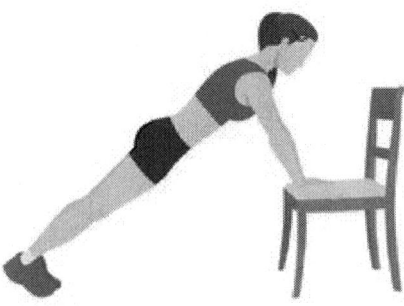

The modified chair yoga plank pose is done like the regular plank but with the support of a chair.

- Return to the starting plank, as you were before the mountain climbers. Hold the side edges of your chair with your hands.

- Extend your legs behind you, keeping a straight back and a neutral spine, toes on the ground, and heels lifted. Shoulders should be aligned with your wrists.

- Engage your core by hardening your abdomen and hold for five seconds. Take deep breaths as you hold.

- Relax and move into a down dog pose where you push your body back, lift your hips and open your legs slightly apart, arms straightened in front of you to hold the chair for support.

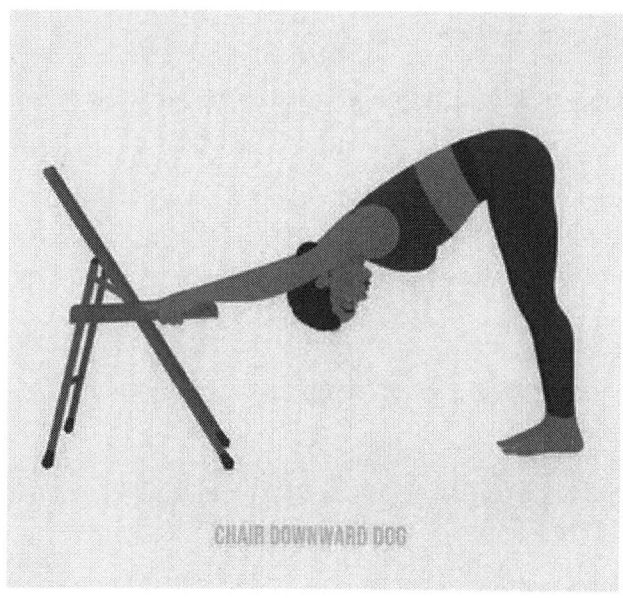

CHAIR DOWNWARD DOG

- Repeat five times.

The other variation of leg raises will strengthen your hip flexors and thighs. To do it:

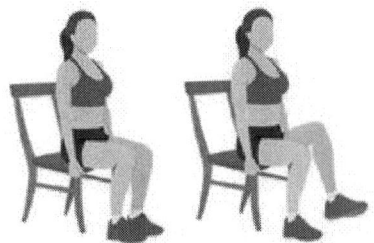

- Sit on your chair, back straight, and knees bent at ninety degrees. Place your hands on the laps.

- Engage your core, lift your right knee slowly towards your chest, and lower it back to the ground. Lift the left knee towards your chest and lower it back to the ground.

- Take deep breaths as you lift your knee and exhale as you lower your knee.

- Engage your core to feel the sensation on your thighs and hips and your core.

- Repeat ten times for each leg.

- After your last repetition, lift your right knee, open it to the side, bring it back to the center, and lower it to the ground.

- Switch the legs and repeat the same moves with your left leg. Match your pace with your breath. Ensure that the movement is just in the hip, not the whole body.

You will feel the sensation on your lower back and upper back, as well as your hips.

Leg Holds

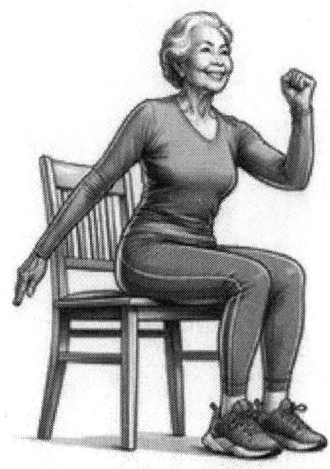

- Sit on the chair, your back slightly away from the chair's back and straight, and your feet on the ground just like you did during leg raises.

- This time, lift both of your legs slightly off the ground and hold them in the air. Take deep breaths as you hold. Ensure a neutral spine the whole time.

- Hold for thirty seconds and relax for two seconds and repeat.

- Repeat four times.

Seated Bicycle Crunches

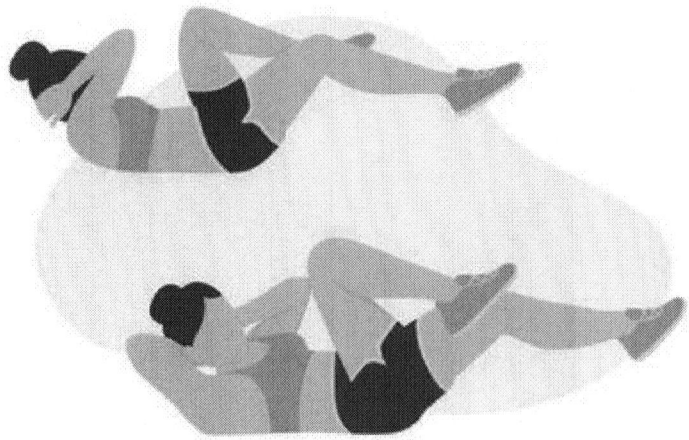

The seated bicycle is a challenging chair yoga pose that strengthens the core and hip flexors.

- Sit tall with a neutral spine and feet on the ground. Lift your hands to bring them towards behind your ears.

- Lift your right foot to twist towards your left leg elbow. Here, you are aiming for that twist at the core and oblique. Even the slightest twist, when done consistently, will help.

- Inhale as you make the twist and exhale as you come back to the center.

- Switch to the left leg. Lift the left knee and twist towards the right-hand elbow as you inhale, then exhale as you return to the center.

- Take your time with the twist, as slow movement is what will help you build strength.

- Complete ten to twenty repetitions for each side.

To make the seated poses even more challenging, hold both your feet off the ground like you would in a boat pose, and try to touch your knees with your right and left elbows interchangeably. Again, slow twisting will be more effective than doing the twists fast.

The seated bicycle crunches can be modified into:

Elbow to Knee Crunch

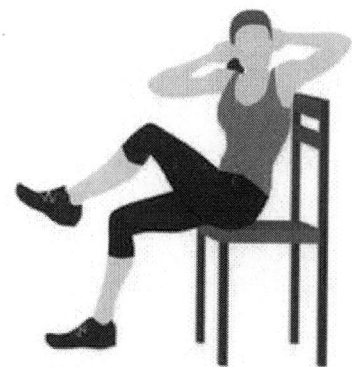

- This time, you will have your hands hanging towards the ground, then lift your right leg knee to meet your left-hand elbow.

- Switch to have your left knee meet your right elbow and continue slowly and in a controlled manner.

- Inhale as you lift your leg to meet your elbow, and exhale as you return your foot to the ground.

- Repeat ten to twenty times for each foot.

The other variation to seated bicycle crunch will involve more engagement of your abdomen and less engagement of your legs.

- Sit tall with a straight back and bring your hands to touch behind your ears.

- Engage your abdomen by squeezing it to harden it, and begin to twist your upper body from the right side to the left as you take deep breaths. Try to maintain no movements on your lower body.

    You will feel the stretch sensation on your obliques and abdomen.

- Do two sets of twenty repetitions.

Forward Bend Variation

- Sit close to the chair's edge and lean forward, maintaining a straight back. Place your hands on your knees. Do not lean too much toward the front.

- Engage your core by squeezing and drawing it in.

- Bend slightly further and then get back to the original bending position. Take deep breaths as you do this.

- Move at a slow, controlled pace allowing you to feel the sensation in your abdominal muscles.

- Repeat twenty times. You can break it into two sets of ten or twenty repetitions, depending on your fitness level.

Back Lean

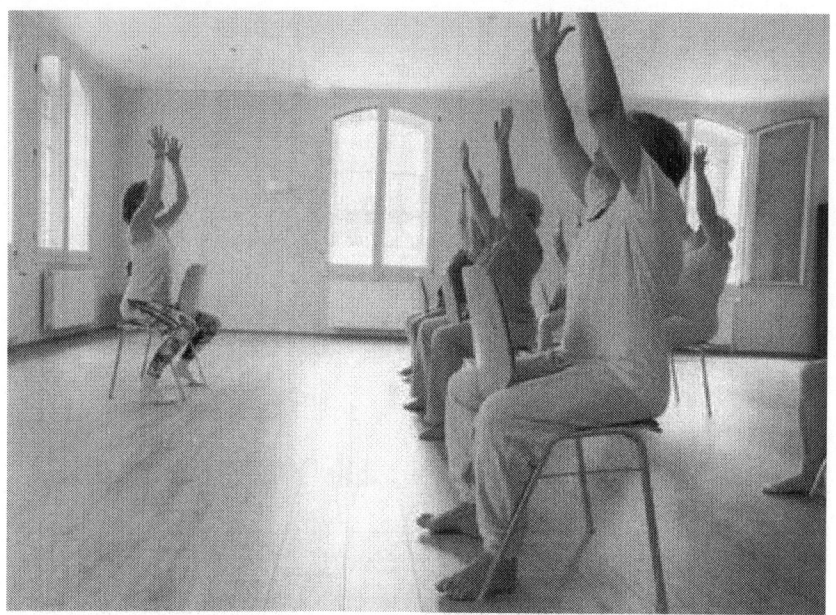

We will move in the opposite direction from the previous forward bends for this pose. This pose looks simple, but it can be very powerful if done right.

- Sit tall at the edge of your chair, with your back nice and straight. Lean back to touch the chair with your back and engage your abdomen by squeezing it in and hardening it.

- Stretch your arms parallel to each other over your head and face the ceiling.

- Press your feet to your heel and slowly bring your body to lean forward. Hold for two seconds.

- Round your back to lean back on the chair and continue like that.

- Inhale as you lean forward, and exhale as you lean backward.

- Move at a slow pace to repeat twenty repetitions.

Seated leg lifts and holds

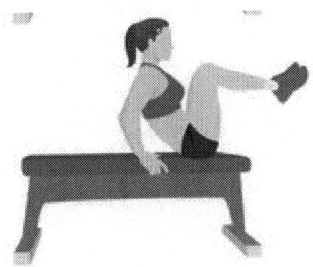

- Sit close to the edge of your chair, just like in back leans.

- Rest your back on the chair and grab the chair by the sides for extra support.

- Harden your abdomen and draw it to engage it and remain that way throughout the pose.

- Lift both legs above the ground to form a V shape, hold for two seconds, gently lower your feet to the ground, and lift again without stopping.

- Repeat ten to twenty times, depending on your level of comfort.

- On your last repetition, lift your legs and hold for five to ten seconds for that final stretch on your core.

Seated Oblique Crunches

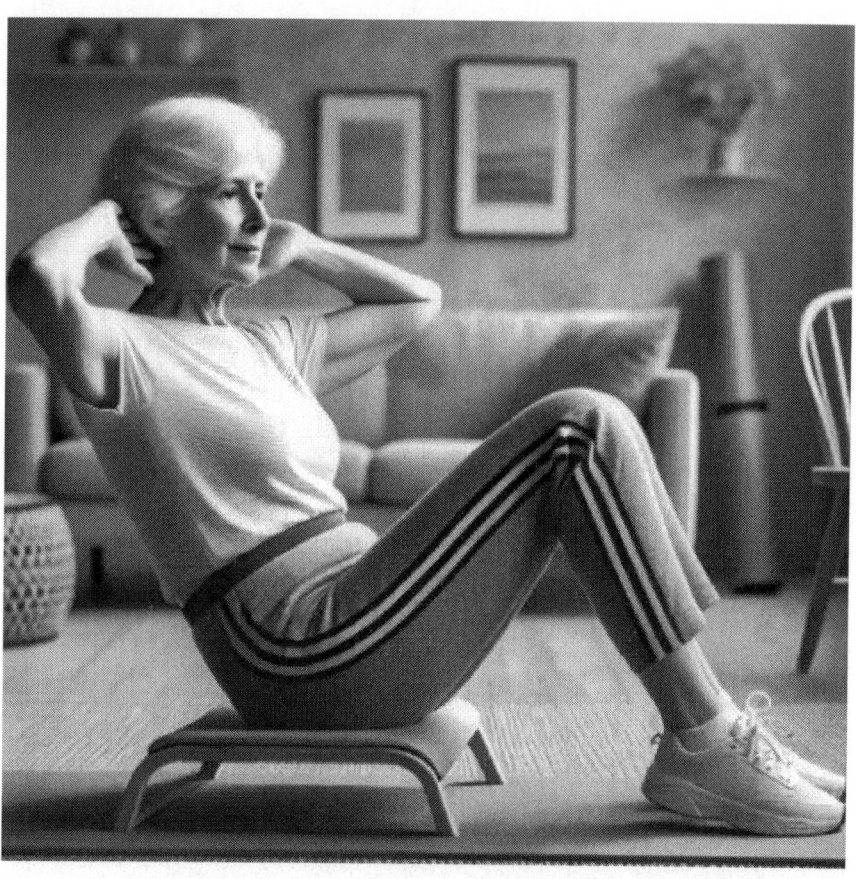

- Sit steady on your chair with a straight back.

- Stretch your arms straight in front of you at chest level, then bend them towards you at the elbow to a 90-degree angle.

- With your arms bent like that, move them to the side to open your chest. Keep your elbows in alignment to your shoulders in a surrender pose.

- Open your legs to the sides, knees over the ankles, and maintain a straight back.

- Inhale and exhale as you lift your right foot, lower your right elbow to meet the right knee, and then inhale back up.

- Switch sides, inhale to lift your left foot, and lower your left elbow to meet the knee, and exhale back up.

This pose works the obliques.

Lift according to your fitness level and aim to feel that stretch on your obliques.

Repeat ten to twenty times for each side.

Core Twist

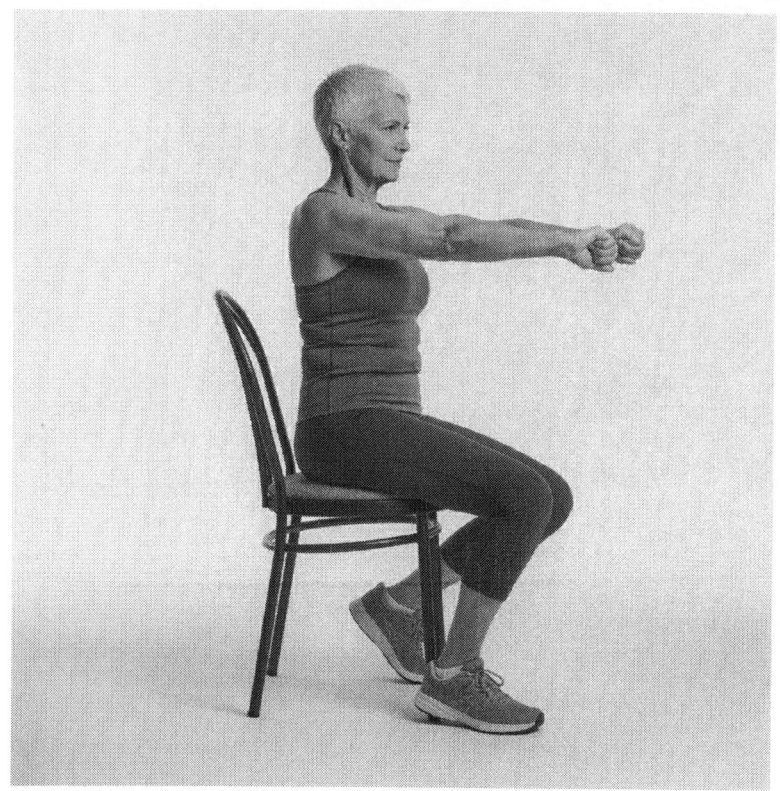

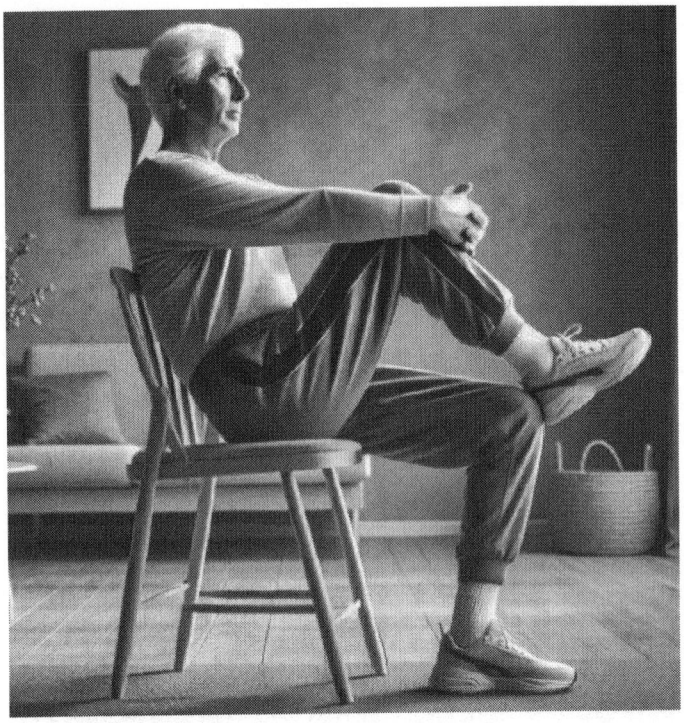

- After your last repetition doing the oblique crunches, release your arms and bring them to your knees. Hold your knees and engage your core by squeezing and drawing it in.

- Drop your right shoulder towards your opposite knee to twist the core. Inhale as you drop towards the knee and exhale as you move back to the center.

- Now drop the left shoulder towards your right knee as you inhale.

- Repeat ten to twenty times for each side.

Chapter 7: Cool Down Chair Yoga Poses

You should spend at least ten seconds on each of these cool-downs.

Cooldowns will allow your body temperature, and heart rate to relax to normal, as well as clear lactic acid from the muscles accumulated during the session.

Cooldowns for Shoulders

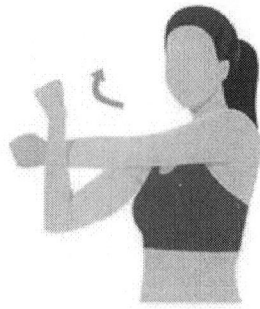

- Hold your left hand's wrist with the back of your left palm, and pull it towards you. Switch hands and repeat with the other hand.

Cool down for arms

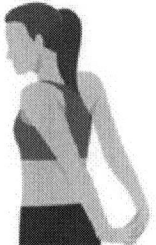

- Bring your hands behind your back. The back of your palms should touch your lower back. While maintaining a straight back, try to move your elbows forward. Hold for two seconds, relax and repeat.

Cool down for the neck

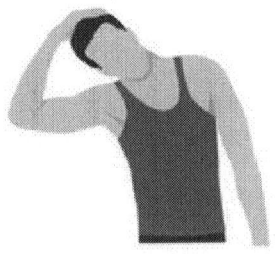

- Sit tall with a straight back. Bend your head towards the left side. Take your left hand and pull your head gently to your shoulder, allowing yourself to feel that stretch, and repeat with the right side.

- After that, slowly lift both arms towards the ceiling with straight fingers.

- Maintain a straight back. Hold for five seconds.

Conclusion

Chair Yoga is amazing proof that you can still work towards staying fit even when life brings limitations such as age, injuries, or limited mobility.

Choose any of the above poses provided in this book to workout every day or at least with consistency, and within no time, you will start reaping the fruits of your efforts.

You will be flexible, stronger, healthier, and happier.

Happy Yoga!

PS: I'd like your feedback. If you are happy with this book, please leave a review on Amazon.

Please leave a review for this book on Amazon by visiting the page below:

https://amzn.to/2VMR5qr

Printed in Great Britain
by Amazon